D1356892

Practical Guide to
Modern Hematology
Analyzers

Practical Guide to Modern Hematology Analyzers

Warren Groner

Center for Laboratory Technology Inc.,
New York, USA

Elkin Simson

Long Island Jewish Medical Center,
The Long Island Campus for the
Albert Einstein College of Medicine,
New York, USA

JOHN WILEY & SONS
Chichester · New York · Brisbane · Toronto · Singapore

Other Wiley Editorial Offices

John Wiley & Sons, Inc., 605 Third Avenue,
New York, NY 10158-0012, USA

Jacaranda Wiley Ltd., 33 Park Road, Milton,
Queensland 4064, Australia

John Wiley & Sons (Canada) Ltd, 22 Worcester Road,
Rexdale, Ontario M9W 1L1, Canada

John Wiley & Sons (SEA) Pte Ltd, 37 Jalan Pemimpin #05–04
Block B, Union Industrial Building, Singapore 2057

Library of Congress Cataloging-in-Publication Data

Groner, Warren.
    Practical guide to modern hematology analyzers / Warren Groner and
Elkin Simson.
        p.   cm.
    Includes bibliographical references and index.
    ISBN 0 471 95712 7
    1. Hematology—Equipment and supplies.   I. Simson, Elkin.
II. Title.
    [DNLM: 1. Leukocyte Count—instrumentation.   2. Pathology,
Clinical—instrumentation.   3. Autoanalysis—instrumentation.
4. Pathology, Clinical—organization & administration.   QY 26 G876p
1995]
RB45.G67   1995
616.07′561′028—dc20
DNLM/DLC
for Library of Congress   95-3302
                                                                    CIP

British Library Cataloguing in Publication Data

A catalogue record for this book is available from the British Library

ISBN 0 471 95712 7

Typeset in 10/12pt Century Schoolbook by Acorn Bookwork, Salisbury, Wilts
Printed and bound in Great Britain by Bookcraft (Bath) Ltd, Midsomer Norton, Avon

Contents

Preface

There has been a slow revolution in the practice of laboratory hematology occurring over the past several years. The seeds of this revolution were planted in the early 1970s with attempts to automate the leukocyte differential, which was then perceived as the last "routine test" still performed manually. Several automated differential counters were developed in this period but none achieved either the technical goal of replacing the trained morphologist or commercial success. However, some of the technology developed for automating the white blood cell differential provided the ability to extend greatly the capability of the "ordinary" cell counter. These modern hematology analyzers are now transforming the practices of hematology laboratories worldwide. Hematology analyzers are essentially cell counters with the ability to measure a variety of characteristics of the cells being counted. Thus, the cell counters are able to both classify and count different cell types. Highly precise counts of the five sub-classes of mature white blood cell are obtained automatically along with the traditional complete blood count, eliminating the need for a microscopic evaluation of the peripheral blood film except for samples which are flagged as abnormal. This has resulted in substantial cost savings in the routine hematology laboratory. In addition, it has substituted a precise objective result based on a relatively low resolution cell counter for the subjective and imprecise visual differential based on examination of 100 or 200 cells.

Commercial instruments are now available from at least five different manufacturers which employ various methods for identifying and classifying the white blood cell. There have been several reports of instrument performance which relate the results to a reference manual differential as defined by the National Committee for Clinical Laboratory Standards (NCCLS) in H20-A and show satisfactory agreement for normal and quantitatively abnormal specimens. However, due to the lack of suitable material there is still limited data from interlaboratory trials. Thus, it is not readily known how well clinical results obtained by repeated sampling of an individual specimen in different laboratories would agree or how easily the results could be used to determine abnormality if the ordering physician was not aware of which method was in use.

The introduction of these devices into the hematology laboratory has also provided a challenge for the laboratory director and/or manager. The modern cell counter provides significant additional information. Some of this information overlaps what has been traditionally obtained at the microscope but does not completely replace it, while some of it is new and of questionable clinical benefit. There is clearly an opportunity to both reduce the cost of laboratory operation and/or improve the quality of service. However, there does not exist a clear tutorial on how to approach the problem practically. Consequently, issues of adjusting laboratory workflow, developing effective quality control procedures, and reporting results to the requesting clinician are being developed by individual laboratories.

It was the authors' intention to address these issues by developing a guide for laboratorians (pathologists, laboratory managers and technologists). It was clear to us that given the wide diversity of needs, specimens, laboratory practices, regulations etc., there was no opportunity to be pedantic. Therefore, we took as our aim to present the subject in as unified a manner as possible so that readers would be able to apply the material to their situation with a better understanding of the issues and how others have dealt with them.

In this guide we first describe the technology (Chapters 1, 2 and 3) by giving the history of the field, some fundamentals of the various key technologies and a description of how some of the modern cell counters work. In Chapters 4 and 5 we deal with the state of the art regarding the performance of the devices, by summarizing the reported data and sharing results obtained in an extensive evaluation at the laboratories of Long Island Jewish Medical Center. We then look into the problems of integrating the system into the routine laboratory (Chapter 6) and finally do a little crystal ball gazing by examining how some of the current research concepts might affect the hematology laboratory of the future (Chapter 7).

We wish to express our gratitude to several individuals who have cooperated by providing data on some of the modern systems. Although we have listed our thanks for their organizations separately we are much indebted to William Canfield of Bayer Diagnostics, Marijane Blunk of Roche Diagnostics, Naomi Culp of Sysmex, Luc Van Hove of Abbott Diagnostics and William Burton of Coulter.

We would also especially like to acknowledge the contribution of our wives who provided encouragement throughout the project in spite of the many hours of companionship they lost as a result of it.

Warren Groner
Elkin Simson

Lake Success, NY, 1995

Acknowledgements

We wish to acknowledge the information provided by the following companies which was invaluable in preparing this book.

Abbott Diagnostics Division,
  Abbott Park, IL, USA

Bayer Diagnostics,
  Tarrytown, NY, USA

Becton Dickinson
  Cellular Imaging Systems,
  San Jose, CA, USA

Chemunex S.A.
  Maisons-Alfort, France

CompuCyte Corp.
  Cambridge, MA, USA

Coulter Corporation,
  Miami, FL, USA

International Medical Imaging, Inc.,
  Palm Beach Gardens, FL, USA

International Remote Imaging Systems Inc.,
  Chatsworth, CA, USA

Roche Diagnostic Systems,
  Brancheburg, NJ, USA

Sysmex Inc.,
  McGraw Park, IL, USA

TOA Medical Electronics Co, Ltd.,
  Kobe, Japan

Chapter 1

History of Cell Counting

INTRODUCTION AND OVERVIEW

Before beginning the discussion and analysis of modern cell counting systems, it is interesting to review the history of the field of cell counting. The history of blood cell analysis can be divided into roughly four phases:

1. Discovery.
2. Application.
3. Consolidation.
4. Rediscovery.

DISCOVERY (1642–1881)

The first phase, which we shall call discovery, began when Leeuwenhook first noted the cells of the blood in 1642, and continued for more than 200 years. It was marked by a series of observations which enabled blood cells to be placed in increasingly refined categories. Notable events included:

- The discovery of platelets by Donne, in 1842 (Donne, 1842) and their enumeration by Hayem in 1875 (Hayem and Nacket, 1875).
- The differentiation between lymphocytes and granulocytes by size recognized by Gulliver as early as 1846 and the enumeration of white blood cells (WBC) by hemocytometry (Malassez, 1874).

The discovery phase was essentially completed with the application of the aniline dyes of Paul Ehrlich (Ehrlich, 1879–80) at the end of the 19th century.

Practical Guide to Modern Hematology Analyzers. W. Groner and E. Simson
© 1995 John Wiley & Sons Ltd

Progress during this discovery phase was principally controlled by the development of the field of optics, which was needed in order to magnify and differentiate the elements of the blood, and by improvement of the stain technology. The stains were used to mark the blood cells and their internal structure, thereby providing the means to differentiate the cells on the basis of their appearance.

APPLICATION (1881–1950)

In the second phase, which we have called application, the microscopic observations and the quantification of the cellular elements of the blood were related to clinical phenomena. This phase began at the turn of the 20th century and was marked by the establishment of relationships between microscopic observation and clinical status. Important discoveries during this phase were:

- Differentiation of the band cell and relating the morphology of neutrophils to infection and inflammation (Arneth, 1904; Schilling, 1929).
- The classification of anemias based on volume and hemoglobin content of red cells (Wintrobe, 1934).
- Defining the function of platelets.
- A detailed classification of leukemias on the basis of morphology (Bennett, 1976).

Most of these applications were based only upon observation with the cause and effect remaining to be established. However, with repeated observation the meaning became accepted and clinicians found that a careful microscopic review of the peripheral blood film added significant value to the clinical history and physical examination, aiding in the diagnosis of disease.

Thus, at the end of the second phase (1950) clinical utility for the complete blood count had been established and this test was ordered routinely on a large number of patients for the purpose of discovering and diagnosing disease as well as for following specific therapies. Principally these tests were performed at the microscope and typically by laboratory scientists who reported the results to the clinician in terms of a series of numbers representing the concentrations of the various cell types, plus qualitative comments on the appearance of the cells.

CONSOLIDATION (1951–1965)

The third phase, which we shall call consolidation, was marked by the automation of the elements of the complete blood count. In this phase, which began in the middle of the 20th century, the principal advances were not in discovery of new cells or cell classifications nor in clinical relevance, but in automation technology and cost reduction. The principal results of this phase were to eliminate a good deal of tedious microscopy in favor of the cell counting machines which are the subject of this book. Thus, the detailed history of this phase is of significance to our purpose and will be considered exclusively in the next section.

REDISCOVERY (1965 TO PRESENT TIME)

The fourth phase, rediscovery, was initiated in the 1960s and continues today. In this phase the focus is on observing with more specific chemistries the molecular structure of the cells and hopefully from this detail completing the causality bridge by which what is observed microscopically at the cellular level in blood can be linked to what is found clinically.

The rediscovery phase began with the elucidation of the specific enzymes within the leukocytes which provided an alternative for classification. Subsequently, specific receptors were found on the surface of lymphocytes allowing their sub-classification along functional lines as well as differentiating among cells which appear similar under the microscope with traditional stains. In this period functional relevance and the functional characteristics of the cells were demonstrated; first, through the use of enzymes (Yam *et al.*, 1971), then, through the use of monoclonal antibodies (Kohler and Milstein, 1975), and finally, through the use of nucleic acid probes (Bauman, 1980).

EARLY HISTORY OF CELL COUNTING TECHNOLOGY

In this section we will begin to deal more thoroughly with the history and the development of the technology which was ultimately applied to quantification of the formed elements of the blood and used in the cell counting machines developed during the consolidation phase described above.

EARLY CELL COUNTERS

The first attempts to enumerate the cells in blood followed closely upon their discovery in the 17th century by Leeuwenhook, who himself counted, with his first microscope, the number of chicken erythrocytes pulled into a glass capillary tube with graduation marks of measured dimension. This general microscopic technique of counting the number of cells in a transparent chamber of measured dimension developed gradually over two centuries with improvements in the microscope and in the design of "counting chambers". In the 19th century, techniques for accurately diluting the blood sample before counting were introduced, allowing more latitude in the design of counting chambers. This resulted in easier and more accurate counting using a shallow rectangular chamber (hematocytometer) with a thin cover glass (designed by Burker, 1905), into which the diluted blood was injected. This basic design, with ruling superimposed, is still employed when manual microscopic cell counts are done.

In the 20th century, with advances in electronics and electro-optics, several attempts to further simplify blood cell counting were made. Moldavan (1934) described an electric procedure by which cells in a dilute erythrocyte suspension were counted individually by a photoelectric device. Because of imperfections in the photoelectric devices of the time, this first attempt in automated erythrocyte counting failed. However, later several automated blood cell counters, based on the same design, were successfully completed.

Around 1945 another method was described with which the concentration of erythrocytes in blood could be determined optically, not by counting individual cells but indirectly by using turbidimetry. The method was further studied and improved upon, resulting in a suitable instrument shown schematically in Figure 1.1. In this instrument, since erythrocytes are not counted one-by-one, the instrument has to be calibrated against the cell reference preparation, or an artificial standard.

In the same decade yet another instrument was described in which erythrocytes could be counted automatically by means of photoelectric spot-scanning of a thin layer of diluted blood sample. In this approach the manual counting chamber technique described above is automated. The microscopist is replaced by a photomultiplier and an electronic counting unit, while the counting chamber is moved by a motor driven system. An instrument based on this principle is the Casella counter shown in Figure 1.2. This technique was also developed further (Langencrantz, 1950) and in later more sophisticated instruments based on flying spot-scanning, special measures were taken to compensate for the errors caused by overlap of cells or irregularities of cell shape (Hodkinson, 1953).

In 1953 a photoelectric counting method was described in which blood cells were forced to pass through an optical detection station in a thin thread of fluid. This procedure reduced the chances of overlapping of blood cells, and cells could be counted one-by-one with a stationary detector. The EEL counter shown in Figure 1.3 is an instrument based on this principle. However, because of the frequent clogging of the long thin capillary through which the blood has to flow, this instrument was rarely used.

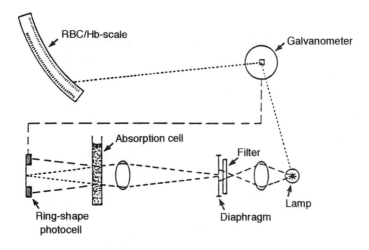

RBC/Hb-scale

Galvanometer

Absorption cell

Filter

Lamp

Ring-shape
photocell

Diaphragm

Figure 1.1   Schematic diagram of a device according to Kleine's light-
scattering method. The intensity of light scattered onto the ring-shaped
photodetector (photocell) is taken as proportional to the concentration of cells in
the absorption cell. From Groner (1970) with permission

In 1956 Coulter discovered another principle for detecting red blood
cells and introduced an automated blood cell counter which made use of
the lesser conductivity of erythrocytes in comparison with that of the
diluting fluid. In Coulter's instrument blood cells suspended in an electrolyte solution are induced to flow through an electric field in a relatively short small orifice drilled in thin sapphire. The electric field in
and surrounding this orifice is the sensing portion of the instrument.
Because of the small dimensions of the sensing portion (also called the
detector), diluted blood cells are readily detected and counted more or
less one-by-one without the high frequency of clogging. This technique
has been extensively developed and serves as the basis for most
modern cell counters. It is alternatively called the "Coulter principle" or
the aperture impedance cell counting method. The first analyzer was
the Model A. This was followed by a series of single channel analyzers
distributed by the Coulter Instrument Company, models B, F, Fn etc.
An important feature of all these analyzers was that they aspirated,
under mercury manometer control, an accurate volume of blood. Today
this type of counter is represented by the coulter ZBI. Cell counters of
this class have been recommended by the International Committee for
Standardization in Hematology (ICSH) as "reference methods" for cell
counting and cell counts obtained with them are used by most manufacturers as the reference counts when assigning red cell and white cell
counts to calibrators and controls.

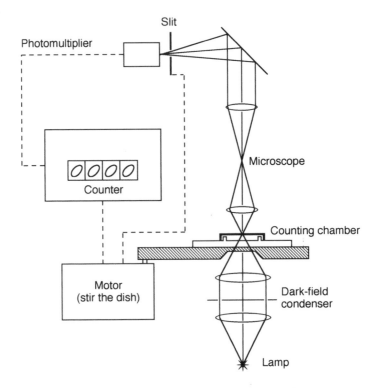

Slit

Photomultiplier

Microscope

Counter

Counting chamber

Motor
(stir the dish)

Dark-field
condenser

Lamp

Figure 1.2 Early cell counter by Casella, using a photo-electric spot scanning method. From Groner (1990) with permission

EARLY CELL SIZING

Measurement of cell size was also initiated by Van Leeuwenhook's invention of the microscope. However, it was not until 1718 that Jurin accurately established the diameter of the human red cell (Jurin, 1718). As with cell counting, measurement of cell size was performed visually until the 20th century. The magnified images of cells (usually flattened in a dried film of blood) were compared to a known dimension by "calibrating the microscope".

Early in the 20th century centrifugation techniques were applied to whole blood, enabling quantitation of the cellular fraction of the blood or a measurement of the packed cell volume (Wintrobe, 1929). Combining this result with the red cell count a red cell index was defined which measured the red cell size indirectly. That is the:

Mean cell volume (MCV) = packed red cell volume fraction divided by red cell count.

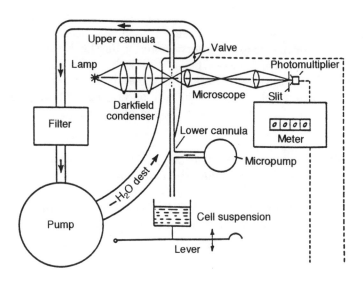

Figure 1.3 Schematic diagram of a device using the photoelectric method of counting cells one at a time. A thin fluid stream containing the cells is passed through a microscope viewing station and each cell's passage is detected by a photomultiplier. From Groner (1990) with permission

The development of Coulter's method of cell counting in the mid-20th century also suggested that cells could be sized simultaneously since the magnitude of the electrical impulse was thought to be proportional to cell volume. Similar arguments were put forth regarding the photo-electric cell counting system and the development of these systems, with a combined purpose of cell counting and cell sizing, has proceeded in parallel over the past three decades.

HEMOGLOBIN DETERMINATION

The earliest attempts to determine the concentration of hemoglobin in the blood include the visual matching of dilutions of whole blood to a liquid color reference by Gowers (1878), Hoppe-Seyler (1883), Sahli (1895), and Haldane (1901). The method of Sahli, in which the blood sample is mixed with hydrochloric acid to obtain acid hematin, is still used frequently. In development of this technique it was found simpler and more quantitative to determine the color through the use of colori-meters and/or spectrophotometer. However, the spectral content of the various forms of hemoglobin precluded the choice of "a good wave-length" at which to measure unless the hemoglobin was first converted to a single stable form. The determination of hemoglobin as cyanmethemoglobin or hemiglobincyanide (HiCN) was introduced by Stahe in 1920 (Stahe, 1920). The hemiglobincyanide method has been studied extensively and has been accepted internationally as the reference method for hemoglobin determination (ICSH, 1978). In a parallel manner to that described above, the measurement of hemoglobin can be combined with the red blood cell count to obtain additional cell indices which indirectly measure the properties of the red blood cells.

That is:

Mean cell hemoglobin concentration (MCHC) = blood hemoglobin concentration divided by packed red cell volume.

Mean cell hemoglobin content (MCH) = blood hemoglobin concentration divided by the red blood cell count.

EARLY MULTIPARAMETER CELL COUNTERS

The first instrument to automate the performance of more than one cell count on a single sample was the SMA 4A-7A introduced by Technicon in 1965. In this instrument, which is shown schematically in Figure 1.4, each sample of blood was divided and diluted using a continuous flow technology which was proprietary to Technicon. The cells in the sample were then counted individually with a photoelectric detector in two passes through a single narrow flow cell. The first pass occurred without the hemolysis of the red blood cells and determined the red blood cell count. The second pass occurred after lysis to determine the WBC count. The hemoglobin was determined in a separate and parallel channel after hemolysis of the red blood cells and conversion of the hemoglobin to cyanmethemoglobin. Determination of the packed cell volume (hematocrit) in the SMA 4A-7A was made by detecting the electrical conductivity of the whole blood. It had previously been shown that an approximately linear inverse relationship existed between the volume conductivity of the whole blood and the packed cell volume (a sort of macroscopic application of the Coulter principle). The red cell indices were then calculated. The instrument produced a seven parameter complete blood count (CBC) on each specimen and operated at a throughput rate of 30 samples per hour.

Although the general concept of combining the analyses in a single instrument was well conceived, the implementation of Technicon's instrument left a great deal to be desired, limiting the proliferation of this device. Of most concern was the accuracy of the packed cell volume derived by the electrical conductivity. A second and more practical concern was the instability of dilution using the Technicon continuous

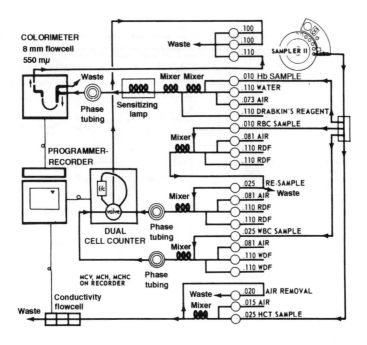

Figure 1.4   Flow diagram of the SMA 4A-7A (courtesy of Bayer Diagnostics, Tarrytown, NY, USA)

flow method. This required that the instrument be periodically recalibrated.

The widespread use of a combined CBC machine was only achieved when Coulter introduced the Model S instrument in 1968. In this instrument the sample was divided via a "blood sampling valve" and diluted into two glass reaction chambers. In one chamber the red blood cells were hemolyzed. Samples from each chamber were passed through electrical counting apertures (Coulter principle) to determine the red blood cell count and the white blood cell count. Hemoglobin was determined by the optical absorption in the white blood cell count reaction chamber without conversion to cyanmethemoglobin. The mean cell volume was calculated from the average signal size in the red blood cell counting aperture. The packed cell volume, mean cell hemoglobin and mean cell hemoglobin concentration were then calculated to produce a seven parameter CBC. Samples were fed into the analyzer manually. A maximum throughput rate of almost 100 samples per hour was possible. The instrument was easy to operate and reliable. Further, the dilution stability achieved with the "blood sampling valve" and reaction chambers allowed for constancy of calibration. By the early 1970s the

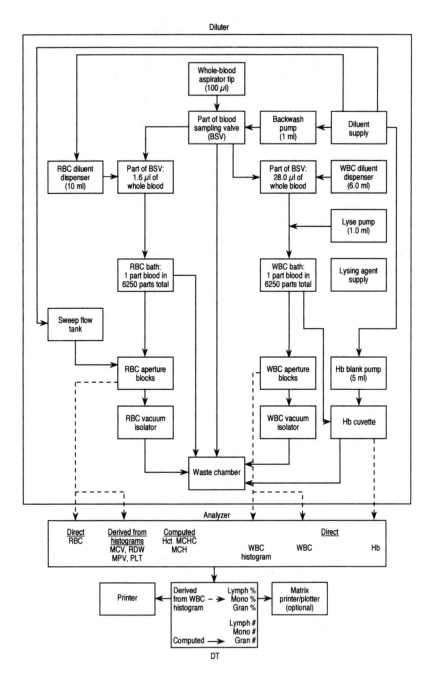

Figure 1.5 Schematic diagram of the Coulter Model S Plus IV cell counter
(courtesy of Coulter Corporation, Hialeah, FL, USA)

Model S had essentially revolutionized the hematology laboratory, consolidating the routine testing into two workstations: the automated CBC (now defined as seven parameters) and the remainder, typically called the WBC differential, which was still performed microscopically. Platelet counts were performed infrequently, using a microscopic manual method in which platelets were counted in a hemocytometer chamber.

In 1970 Technicon introduced the Hemalog-8 instrument which added the platelet count to the seven parameter automated CBC. This instrument also used the continuous flow approach to sample division and dilution. Platelets were counted in an additional parallel counting channel by photoelectric means after hemolysis of the red blood cells in a strong solution of urea. However, unlike its predecessor, the SMA 4A-7A, the packed cell volume was determined on the Hemalog-8 system by automation of the centrifugal packing of the red cells followed by a photoelectric scan which registered the cell/plasma interface. The system used an automated sampler and worked initially at a throughput of 60 samples per hour. In 1974 the company introduced a higher speed version at 90 samples per hour. Since the continuous flow dilution method was employed, periodic calibration was still required.

Again, although the introduction and inclusion of the platelet count as part of the CBC was well received, the implementation of the Technicon instrument fell short and it did not achieve widespread use principally due to the lack of reliability of the automated centrifuge and the requirement for periodic calibration.

The next major advance was made when Coulter introduced the S Plus series which added the platelet count to their automated CBC instrument. In this instrument, which was introduced in 1980, the platelet count was derived simultaneously in the red blood cell counting aperture by discriminating between platelets and red blood cells on the basis of signal size. As with the predecessor Coulter Model S, the mean cell volume was determined by the average signal height of the red blood cells and the packed cell volume calculated by multiplication with the red count. Mean cell hemoglobin and mean cell hemoglobin concentration were calculated from the hemoglobin determination and the red blood cell count and the packed cell volume PCV determination respectively. The Coulter Model S Plus operated manually at a throughput approaching 100 samples per hour. A subsequent model, the S Plus II, added further parameters to the reported results of the automated CBC. In addition to the platelet count, four other parameters were added:

1. The red cell distribution width, which was defined as the spread (coefficient of variation) of the red cell signal distribution.

2. The mean platelet volume, which was defined in analogy to the mean red cell volume by averaging the signal heights from the platelets.
3. The lymphocyte percentage, which was defined by discriminating the signal size in the white cell counting aperture between small cells and large cells and defining the small cells as lymphocytes.
4. The lymphocyte count, which was obtained by multiplying the lymphocyte percentage by the total white cell count.

The Coulter S Plus II also included histogram analysis of the cell size distribution for each of the cell types: white blood cells, red blood cells and platelets.

The next major advance in consolidation of cell counting was also made by Coulter with the introduction of the Coulter S Plus IV (shown schematically in Figure 1.5) system in 1983. In the S Plus IV system additional discrimination on the basis of size was made for the white blood cell signal distribution. White cells were classified into three categories: lymphocytes, monocytes and granulocytes. In addition, another platelet parameter was added; The platelet distribution width derived in analogy with the red cell distribution width which was introduced with the Coulter Model S Plus II.

AUTOMATION OF THE LEUKOCYTE DIFFERENTIAL

The consolidation of cell counting which occurred in the 1960s, together with parallel developments of automation in the clinical chemistry laboratory, focused attention on the microscopic determination of the unautomated portion of the CBC, which was loosely called the white blood cell differential count. This description, however, was not completely accurate since the microscopic process included, in addition to counting and classifying some 100 leukocytes, the subjective analysis of the stained cells (including the red blood cells and platelets).

Since this process was tedious and time consuming and represented the last unautomated routine test, intense activity was initiated during the 1970s in attempts to automate the leukocyte differential count. These attempts followed two different technology approaches. In one, a direct attempt was made to automate the microscopic procedure using pattern recognition and automated image analysis of a stained blood film. In the other, called flow systems, an attempt was made to use the general principles of automated cell counting applied to cells after tagging them with specific stains. Figure 1.6 summarizes the history of these developments from 1950 to 1980.

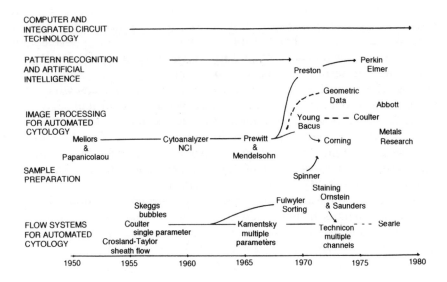

Figure 1.6 Historical development of automated differential systems illustrating the parallel development of image processing and flow technologies, and supporting advances in sample preparation, computer and integrated circuit technology, and pattern recognition. From Bacus (1978) with permission

IMAGE PROCESSING

One of the first achievements in automated image processing was that of Mellors and Papanicolaou in 1952 (Mellors *et al.*, 1952). This same Papanicolaou, who had developed the Pap stain for cervical cytology, was also investigating an instrument which was intended to automatically screen cervical smears based on fluorescent staining. He and Mellors discovered that cancer cells often emitted more fluorescence per unit area than normal cells and constructed a photoelectric scanner which automatically measured the signals of nuclear fluorescence. It turned out that this single parameter did not have enough discriminating power to screen for cervical cancer and the instrument was not pursued further. However, the principle of organizing the signals resulting from a photoelectric scan of a cell by features had been established.

The next development in image processing occurred in the late 1950s and early 1960s. This was the Cytoanalyzer project sponsored by the USA National Cancer Institute, also for the purpose of screening cervical smears for the detection of abnormal cells. It was constructed to scan a slide and measure two parameters, nuclear size and nuclear density. It actually made several feature measurements on all large dense objects in the field and classified these objects according to a multidimensional decision space defined by these features. The Cytoanalyzer was an attempt ahead of its time with respect to the development of companion technologies of pattern recognition, artificial intelligence and computer technology. It did not work because the logic was not capable of telling the difference between large dense areas which were the cervical cell nuclei and those which were clumped leukocytes, etc. Nevertheless, this work stimulated Prewitt and Mendelsohn (1966) who constructed a research oriented device called the Cydac Scanning Microscope System. This system was primarily used for the analysis of chromosomes. However, one of the first studies with the equipment involved the feasibility of blood cell classification.

As indicated in Figure 1.6, research proceeded with other imaging processing systems in blood cell classification, which took place in the late 1960s and early 1970s. Significant contributions were made by Ingram and Preston (1970), Young (1969), and Bacus (1971). By 1973 algorithms to classify at least six major normal white blood cell categories including segmented and banded neutrophils, lymphocytes, monocytes, eosinophils and basophils were available together with means of evaluating performance results.

These research results began to look so promising that commercial developments aimed at automating the WBC differential were initiated. The research results were incorporated into clinical laboratory instruments which would automatically classify blood cells in a rapid, routine, and reliable fashion. One of the first instruments developed during this period was the Larc manufactured by Corning Glass and reported at the International Congress of Hematology in 1972. These were the first reports in the scientific literature of a routinely working automated WBC differential instrument in the hematology laboratory. Figure 1.7 indicates a condensed classification of the flow logic for the Larc instrument.

Subsequent to the development of the Larc system, additional commercial systems based on image analysis were developed and released by Geometric Data (Hematrak) in 1974, Coulter (Diff-3) in 1974, and Abbott (ADC 500) in 1978.

In spite of the development of several instruments which produced a sub-classification of the mature white blood cells, plus qualitative estimates of red blood cell morphology, and information regarding abnormal nucleated cells, these automated WBC differential instruments never attained the widespread popularity in routine hematology that had been accorded to their companion instrument, the multiparameter cell counters. The reason for this lack of success lay in the benefit versus cost analysis.

The multiparameter cell counters provided complete automation

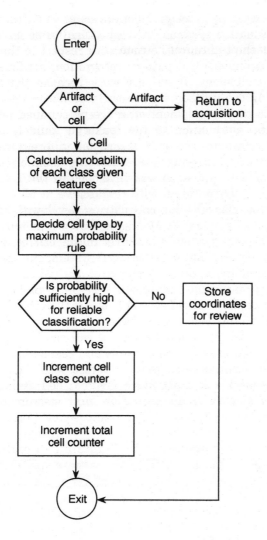

Figure 1.7 Classification flow logic for the Larc differential counter. From Bacus (1978) with permission

(from incoming sample to reported results) and completely eliminated the need for performing at least two microscopic cell counts as well as the hemoglobin and packed cell volume determinations. On the other hand, the more expensive image processing instruments only automated the microscopic examination of the Wright stained blood film. The preparation and staining of the blood film were still done manually (often to more exacting specifications than for visual observation).

Further, since most hematology laboratories at that time did not have laboratory information systems, the results had to be manually entered on reports from the cell counter output.

FLOW METHODS

In parallel with the development of image processing systems, another approach to the automation of the leukocyte differential was made using enzyme cytochemistry as a means for differentiating the white blood cells and then counting and classifying them in an optical cell counting system. This approach was developed by the Technicon Instrument Company in collaboration with researchers at Mount Sinai School of Medicine. Basic classification chemistries, developed and reported by Ornstein and Ansley (1974) at Mount Sinai, were automated using the continuous flow methodology of the Technicon cell counting systems. The first resulting automated differential system, the Hemalog-D, was released commercially in 1974 (Mansberg *et al.*, 1974). Figure 1.8 shows a schematic diagram of the Hemalog-D system. In this system the cells were classified in three parallel channels. In the first channel, myeloperoxidase containing cells were stained by precipitating 4 chloro-1-naphthyl. The resulting differentiation of cell size and color was then used to classify lymphocytes, neutrophils and eosinophils. In the second channel the intracellular nonspecific esterase was used to specifically identify the monocytes at a pH which favored their staining relative to the other granulocytes. Alpha naphthol butyrate was used as a sub-

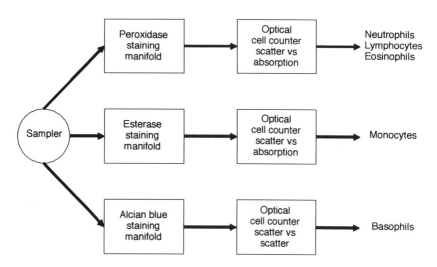

Figure 1.8   Schematic diagram of the Technicon Hemalog-D cytochemical
WBC differential

strate. The third channel specifically classified basophils on the basis of reaction with the Alcian blue stain which had been developed for the accurate counting of basophils visually in counting chambers. The system used automated sampling at 60 samples per hour and completely automated the process. The principal difference between the flow approach and the image recognition approach is that the flow approach classifies a greater number of cells on a smaller number of classification features. In the Hemalog-D, 10 000 cells were classified in each channel thereby achieving high reproducibility for the cell counts.

However, as with the automated differential instruments based on image analysis the use of the flow through differential systems was limited. Thus, even with the greater degree of automation achieved with these instruments, the benefits did not outweigh the costs. In many of the samples microscopic evaluation was still required to complete the report with regard to red blood cell morphology and abnormal cells. Because of the continuous flow technology, frequent recalibration was necessary. Further, the results still had to be manually added to the report form from the multiparameter cell counter. Technicon struggled to improve the benefits, first by increasing the analysis rate to 90 samples per hour (introduced in 1978 as the Hemalog-D90), and second by combining the Hemalog-D system and the Hemalog-8 system with a common sampler. This combination produced the first prototype of the modern multiparameter cell counting system.

THE MODERN MULTIPARAMETER CELL COUNTING SYSTEMS

The first modern multiparameter cell counting system was the Technicon H6000 introduced in 1981. In this system Technicon completed the combination described above by physically combining on a single platform the cell counting technology which it had developed independently for the automated CBC (Hemalog-8) and the automated leukocyte differential (Hemalog-D). Redundant channels were eliminated and the H6000 produced a combined CBC plus five part leukocyte differential at 60 samples per hour. However, commercial success for the H6000 was limited for the same reasons that prevented success of the earlier Technicon cell counters. That is, it was difficult to operate and required periodic calibration. As with previous Technicon hematology instruments, the H6000 demonstrated the value of consolidating hematology testing in a single workstation but failed to achieve commercial success as a result of poor implementation.

The modern multiparameter cell counters, which will be discussed in greater detail in the subsequent chapters of this book, represent exploitation of this advance. The first of the modern systems was the Technicon H*1 system which was launched at the end of 1985. Since that time, additional systems which combine the counting of the traditional automated CBC with white blood cell differentials have been introduced by Coulter, Abbott, TOA and Roche.

REFERENCES

Arneth, J. (1904) *Die neutrophilea weisser Blutkorperchen bei Infections Krankheiten*. G. Fisher, Jena.

Bacus, J.W. (1971) *An Automated Classification of the Peripheral Blood Leukocytes by Means of Digital Image Processing*. Ph.D. Thesis, Univ. of Ill. Med. Ctr.

Bacus, J.W. (1978) The development of automated differential systems. In Koepke, J. (ed.) *Differential Leukocyte Counting*. CAP, Skokie, Ill.

Bauman, J.G.J., Weigant, J. and Van Dujin, P. (1980) Cytochemical hybridisation with fluorochrome labelled DNA. *Exp. Cell Res.* **128**: 485.

Bennett, J.M., Catovsky, D., Daniel M.T. *et al.* (1976) Proposal for the classification of the acute Leukemias. *Br. J. Haematol.* **33**: 451.

Burker, K. (1905) Eine neue Form der Zahlkammer. *Arch. Gesante Physiol. Menschen Tiere*, **107**: 426.

Coulter, W.H. (1956) High speed automatic blood cell counter and cell size analyzer. *Proceedings of the National Electronics Conference* **12**, 1034–40.

Donne, A. (1842) De l'origine des globules du sang, de leur mode de formation et de leur fin. *C.R. Acad. Sci.* **14**: 366–8.

Ehrlich, P. (1879–80) Methodologische Beitrage zur Physiologie und Pathologie der versciedenen Formen der Leukocyten. *Z. Klin. Med.* **1**: 553–60.

Gowers (1878) Meeting Clinical Society of London. *Lancet* **ii**: 882–3.

Groner, W. (1990) Cell counters. In Webster, J. (ed.) *Encyclopedia of Medical Devices*. J. Wiley, New York.

Haldane, J. (1901) The colorimetric determination of haemoglobin. *J. Physiol.* **26**: 497–502.

Hayem, G. and Nacket, A. (1875) Sur un nouveau procede pour compter les globules du sang. *C. R. Acad. Sci.* **80**: 1083–8.

Hodkinson, J.R., (1953) Coincidence and overlap errors in the automatic counting and sizing of particles. *Nature (London)* **171**: 351.

Hoppe-Seyler, F. (1883) *Hanbuch der Physiologisch-und Pathologisch Chemischen Analyse fur Aertzte und Studierende*, pp. 435–40. Hoischwald, Berlin.

ICSH (1978) Recommendations for reference method for haemoglobinometry in human blood and specifications for international haemoglobincyanide reference preparation. *J. Clin. Pathol.* **31**: 139–43.

Ingram, M.L. and Preston, K. Jr. (1970). Automatic analysis of blood cells. *Sci. Am.* **223**: 72–82.

Jurin, J. (1718) An account of some experiments relating to the specific gravity of human blood. *Phil. Trans. R. Soc. London* **361**: 1000.

Kohler, G. and Milstein, C. (1975) Continuous cultures of fused cells secreting antibody of predefined specificity. *Nature* **256**: 495–7

Langercrantz, C. (1950) Photo-electric counting of individual microscopic plant and animal cells. *Nature (London)* **161**: 25.

Malassez, L.C. (1874) Nouvelle methode de numeration des globules rouges et des globules blancs du sang. *Arch. Physiol. norm. path.* (2) **i**: 32–52.

Mansberg, H.P., Saunders, A.M. and Groner, W. (1974) The Hemalog D white cell differential system. *J. Histochem. Cytochem.* **22**: 711.

Mellors, R.C., Glassman, A. and Papanicolaou, G.N. (1952). *Cancer* **5**: 458–68.

Moldavan, A. (1934) Photo-electric technique for the counting of microscopical cells. *Science* **80**: 188–9.

Ornstein, L. and Ansley, H.R. (1974) Spectral matching of classical cytochemistry to automated cytology. *J. Histochem. Cytochem.* **22**: 453–69.

Preston, K. and Norgren, P.E. (1971) US Patent No. 3, 577,267.

Prewitt, J.M.S. and Mendelsohn, M.L. (1966). Analysis of cell images. *Ann. N. Y. Acad. Sci.* **128**: 1035–53.

Sahli, H. (1895) Bestimmung des Hamoglobingehaltes des Blutes. In *Lehbuch der Klinischen Untersuchungsmethoden*, Vol. II, pp. 361–73. Deuticke, Leipzig.

Schilling, V. (1929) *The Blood Picture and its Clinical Significance.* C.V. Mosby, St. Louis, MO.

Stahe, W.C. (1920) A method for the determination of methemoglobin in blood. *J. Biolog. Chem.* **41**: 237–41.

Wintrobe, M.M. (1929) A simple and accurate hematocrit. *J. Lab. Clin. Med.* **15**: 287–289.

Wintrobe, M.M. (1934) Classification of the anaemias on the basis of differences in the size and hemoglobin of the red corpuscles. *Proc. Soc. Exp. Biol. Med.* **27**: 1071.

Yam, L., Li, C. and Crosby, W. (1971) Cytochemical identification of monocytes and granulocytes. *Am. J. Clin. Pathol.* **55**: 283–90.

Young, I. T. (1969) *Automated Leukocyte Recognition.* Ph.D. Thesis, Mass. Inst. Tech.

FURTHER READING

Ansley, H.R. and Ornstein, L. (1973) U.S. Patent No. 3,741,875.

Daland, J. (1891) Ueber das Volumen der roten und weissen Blutkorperchen in Blute des gesunden und kranken Menschen. *Fortsch. Med.* **9**: 87–101.

Dare, A. (1900) A new hemoglobinometer for the examination of undiluted blood. *Philadelphia Med. J.* **6**: 555–60.

Fleischl, E. von (1885) Das Hamometer. *Medizinische Jahrbuch* **15**: 425–33.

Langercrantz, C. (1952) On the theory of counting individual microscopic cells by photoelectric scanning. An improved counting apparatus. *Acta Physiol. Scand.* **26**: 92.

Truk, W. (1907) Ueber den Farbeindex der roten Blutkorperchen. *Munchener Medizinsche Wochenschrift* **54**: 220–32.

Truk, W. (1904) *Vorlesungen uber Klinische Hamatologie.* Braunmuller, Wein.

Vierordt, K. (1852) Zahlungen der Blutkorperchen des Menschen. *Arch. Physiol. Heilkunde* **11**: 546–58.

Wintrobe, M. (1980) *Blood Pure and Eloquent.* McGraw-Hill, New York.

Young, J.Z. and Roberts, F. (1951) A flying spot microscope. *Nature (London)* **167**: 231.

Chapter 2

Technology Fundamentals

INTRODUCTION

Conceptually the objective of a cell counting instrument can be stated simply: determine the number of cells in a given volume by counting them one at a time. However, as we shall see, this problem is more technically challenging than it may appear from the simply stated objective. The challenge for the modern cell counter arises from three general reasons:

1. The characteristics of the blood cells.
2. The volume accounting difficulty.
3. The need to sub-classify the cells.

In the following few paragraphs we will briefly describe the impact of these general problems and then in the rest of the chapter explain how the technology used in cell counters has been developed to address these problems.

THE CHARACTERISTICS OF BLOOD CELLS

The most obvious technical challenges stem directly from the nature of blood, in particular, that the cells are quite small and highly concentrated. These facts produce some technical problems. First, the cells are small and hence they are difficult to detect individually, i.e. to be effective the counting device must be able to discriminate reliably the signals produced by objects with the dimensions of microns from other spurious inputs (typically called background noise). Also since the cells are small, the same detecting device must have a small sensing zone and be able to count one cell at a time, yet be large enough to allow a cell to pass. Secondly, the cells are highly concentrated in whole blood,

Practical Guide to Modern Hematology Analyzers. W. Groner and E. Simson
© 1995 John Wiley & Sons Ltd

hence the space between cells is not large compared to the sensing volume. Thus there is a high probability that a second cell may enter the sensing zone before the previous cell has exited. As a result, two cells may be counted as one. This is called a coincidence, and the resulting counting error called coincidence error. Typically, for human blood specimens the packed cell volume is greater than 25%. Thus, the space between cells is not great enough in undiluted blood to count cells without substantial coincidence error. To deal with this problem a cell counter must use two steps. In the first step the whole blood sample is prepared by dilution so that the cells are reasonably separate (space between cells larger than the cell dimension). In the second step they are caused to pass essentially one at a time through a sensing zone which is sensitive enough to detect their passage. There is an obvious relationship between the first and second steps; that is, the dimensions of the sensing zone determine the amount of dilution required.

VOLUME ACCOUNTING

A second and equally challenging problem is that when the cells are counted and the concentration reported as the number per unit volume, the volume referred to is the original whole blood volume. Thus, all of the steps required to analyze the sample must constantly keep track of the volumes and be able to refer back to the original sample volume. This is the essential difference between a cell counter and a flow cytometer; i.e. the cell counter is a flow cytometer that keeps track of the sample volume.

Volume accounting is a more complex problem than might appear for two reasons: first, the blood is a two phase fluid with a mixture of particles and fluid at different density. Consequently, the homogeneity of the solution is not guaranteed and constant attention must be paid to avoid separations due to settling of the cells or their adherence to surfaces; secondly, as a result of the flexibility and density of the red blood cell, the whole blood is a non-Newtonian fluid and has strange properties in flow. These properties can create inhomogeneity in cell concentration under a variety of flow conditions. For instance, as the blood flows in a cylindrical tube the deformable red cells crowd toward the center of the tube causing an inhomogeneity (Goldsmith and Karino, 1980). Thus, traditional laboratory techniques such as pipetting and aliquotting can distort the original cell volume concentration even when the specimen is well mixed.

The cell counter must perform the required dilutions and any other steps required to prepare the specimen for counting without losing track of the relationship between the cells and the original sample volume. Typically, this problem is addressed by carefully controlling sample and fluid delivery volumes both in absolute and relative terms. However, it is generally not feasible to characterize the volume sufficiently accurately to establish the relationship in manufacture. Therefore, a calibration is typically required to establish the dilution factor for the cell counting channel. Precision of volume delivery is then relied upon to maintain the calibration.

CELL CLASSIFICATION

The third technically challenging issue is that the total count of all cells in the blood, although interesting, has little significance. Medical value is only obtained by counting the cells within a class, i.e. red cells, leukocytes and platelets. The concentrations of the different cell classes differ by orders of magnitude: Typically there are 100 RBC for every WBC and 20 RBC for every platelet. In general, the greater the ability to discriminate between cell classes, the greater the medical utility of the result. In order to sub-classify the cell counts the treatment of the cells prior to cell counting is made more complex. Steps are added (such as lysing the red blood cells) to enhance the cell counter's ability to discriminate between cell classes. In addition, the cell counter itself is made more complex by the requirement not only to count cells, but to classify them accurately. Modern multiparameter cell counters (the subject of this book) typically count the cells of the blood and classify them into (a minimum of eight different categories) three different classes, WBC, RBC and platelets, with five to six types of WBC (neutrophils, lymphocytes, etc.). The classification is done by processing the blood sample in parallel channels and then counting the cells with appropriate discrimination algorithms. In some channels a single cell type is counted after discriminating against noise and other cell types. However, in order to minimize the hardware required, modern counters typically classify two or more types of cell in a single cell counting channel. This greatly complicates the problem of coincidence and detection which were discussed above.

CELL COUNTER FUNDAMENTALS

Before describing the technology employed in specific commercial multiparameter cell counting systems, it is useful to spend a little time on each of the functions involved in cell counting and describe the technical issues that surround it.

As we have seen from the above discussion, a cell counter is characterized by a small sensing zone through which cells diluted from whole blood are caused to flow essentially one at a time and create a signal. These signals are processed to produce results including a cell count, cell classification and cell size distributions. The modern cell counter performs these functions automatically and rapidly using a wide array of technology including: mechanical motions, electronics, optics, chemistry, hydraulics and computer science.

Further, as we shall see when we discuss the commercial systems, the specific applications of these technologies vary between the counters produced by different manufacturers. However, since the inputs (blood samples) and the outputs (hematology parameters) are the same, the technical challenges are similar and unifying concepts can be used to establish an orderly way of describing the technology. In the following sections we will attempt to accomplish this by focusing in turn on the generic aspects of each of a series of fundamental elements and describing the approaches and limitations. In particular we will cover:

1. Detection technology.
2. Fluid transport technology.
3. Signal processing.
4. Cell sizing.
5. Cell identification.
6. Multiple cell classification.

DETECTION TECHNOLOGY

All cell counters detect the presence of a cell as a response to the disturbance made by the cell in passing through a pre-existing electromagnetic field. However, different technologies are employed to create the field and as a result different biophysical properties of the cell are responsible for the creation of the signal. The most striking difference is in the frequency of oscillation of the field. Detection in an essentially static electric field, as invented by Coulter, is traditionally called the aperture impedance or the electrical method, while a field of optical frequency is called the light scatter or optical method.

More recently, it has been found that whereas the signal at low frequency (DC) is principally defined by the cell volume, the electrical signal at higher frequency (RF) is influenced by the internal structure of the cell. This observation has been used to enhance the discrimination capacity of the electrical method.

The following paragraphs describe the essentials of these different techniques.

Electrical method (aperture impedance)

The electrical method of measuring cells is shown diagrammatically in Figure 2.1. Cells diluted from whole blood and suspended in an electro-

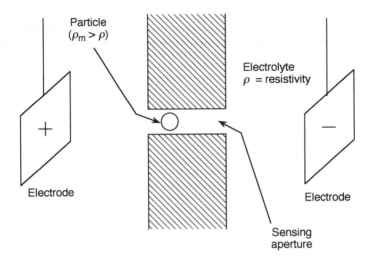

Figure 2.1 Principle of operation for the electrical method of counting cells. From Groner (1988). Reprinted by permission of John Wiley & Sons, Inc.

lyte are caused to flow through a small aperture in an insulator. Electrodes are placed in large baths of electrolytes on either side of the aperture (Coulter, 1956). To a first approximation the aperture may be considered a resistance in a simple circuit governed by Ohm's law. That is, the magnitude of the current is proportional to the applied voltage and inversely proportional to the resistance. Applying Ohm's law for the case when there is no particle in the aperture one obtains for the resistance:

$$R = \frac{V}{I} = \rho(l/a)$$

Where: V is the voltage between the electrodes,
         I is the current flow,
         R is the resistance of the aperture,
         ρ is the resistivity of the electrolyte,
         l is the length of the aperture,
         a is the cross sectional area of the aperture.

When a small particle of much higher resistivity than the electrolyte enters the aperture, it displaces the electrolyte and the resistance of the aperture is increased. The particle acts like a non-conducting hole displacing the conducting electrolyte solution. The altered resistance can be calculated from first principles by considering the details of the geometry within the aperture and summing up (integration) the effects of the conducting volumes (electrolyte) and non-conducting volumes (cells). As an example the case in which the blood cell is modelled by a sphere of infinite resistance has been treated in some detail (Kubitschek, 1960) yielding:

$$\Delta R = Kv(1 + \frac{4}{5} \, x + \frac{843}{1120} \, x^2 + ..)$$

Where:

delta R is the change in current flow,
K is the resistance of the aperture divided by its volume,
v is the volume of the sphere,
x is the ratio of the cross section of the sphere to the cross section of the aperture.

Thus, provided the dimensions of the particle are small relative to the aperture the resulting signal will be linear with the particle volume. Choosing an aperture diameter of 50 μm and maintaining a constant current yields pulses whose peak voltages are linear with the particle's volume (within 5%) from 10 fl to 140 fl.

The size resolution for the aperture impedance detection system is ultimately limited by the ratio of the signal voltage to the fluctuations in detector current (Johnson noise) associated with the aperture resistance. This is called the signal to noise ratio (S/N). The S/N increases as the square root of the ratio between the particle size and the aperture sides. Therefore, extending the range over which the signal size is proportional to the particle size by increasing the aperture dimension can only be done at the expense of size resolution. For the example given (50 μm) the size resolution is approximately 1 fl. It is clear that the aperture diameter is critical in the electrical method. If the aperture is too large, detection of small particles is compromised due to the reduction of signal. If the aperture is too small, the linear range of the size measurement is reduced. In modern hematology systems an aperture of approximately 50 μm is used for counting RBC and platelet, while an aperture of 100 μm is typical for WBC.

In the simple theoretical construct described, the cell was modeled as having a much higher resistance (essentially infinite) than the fluid in which it is suspended. This would seem unreasonable when one considers the case of a red blood cell suspended in isotonic saline. However, if the cell membrane is intact it effectively isolates the cell from the media surrounding it, creating the electrical equivalent of a highly resistant object. Thus, the signal obtained in the aperture impedance method for a red blood cell does not depend on the resistance of the content of the cell as much as the integrity of the insulating membrane. For this reason resealed red cell ghosts (RBC which have been hemolyzed and the membrane repaired) give the same signal as intact red blood cells in the aperture impedance system. There is, however, an indirect effect of the internal constituents of the cell on the signal size. Generally, the content of the cell affects the degree to which the cell is deformed by hydraulic forces while passing through the aperture. This in turn affects the ratio of the cell cross section to that of the aperture (x in the equation above) creating a second order effect on the signal. Thus, the size calibration for a given aperture is not transferable between non-deformable spheres and deformable red blood cells. Consequently different constants must be used to relate signal size to volume for spheres and for cells. The relationship between these calibration constants is called the shape factor.

The simple theoretical model above also assumed that the aperture contents form a cylindrical resistor in which the current density is uniform. Unfortunately, this assumption is not strictly true. Current density is not uniform throughout the aperture, but is significantly higher at the edges of the entrance and exit of the aperture than in the center. Also the electrolyte flow velocity is higher in the center of the aperture than it is at the periphery, according to familiar parabolic laminar flow pattern. Consequently, some particles approach the aperture obliquely and travel close to the wall. These nonaxial particles move more slowly than those that pass through the center. They enter and leave the aperture boundaries through zones of higher current density and may suffer shape distortion as a result of the higher shear forces near the aperture wall. As a result the relationship between signal amplitude and size may be compromised for these non-axial cells resulting in an error in the cell sizing.

There are two practical solutions to the problem of non-axial cells. One is to remove the signals or edit the pulses electronically. This is possible because cells taking a nonaxial path dwell in the effective aperture sensing zone for a longer time than cells taking the axial path. Electronic circuits capable of recognizing this difference and rejecting the longer pulses are called pulse editing circuits. Pulse editing circuits have been used for several years and have proved highly effective. Another solution is provided by confining the particles hydrodynamically to the center of the aperture (sheath flow). This second solution is called hydrodynamic focusing and will be discussed in some detail in the section on fluid transport.

Optical method (light scattering)

In very general terms the light scattering method for measuring cells is shown in Figure 2.2. Light from an optical source propagating in a medium with an index of refraction (n_0) impinges upon the cell which is

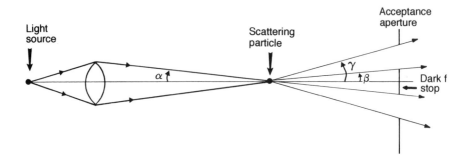

Figure 2.2 Example of the light scattering method for measuring cells. From Groner (1988). Reprinted by permission of John Wiley & Sons, Inc.

characterized by its volume, shape and index of refraction (n_b). The interaction of the incident radiation and the cell produces a scattered wave having intensity which varies with scattering angle. The illumination is blocked by a dark stop and a portion of this scattered wave is collected by an acceptance aperture and falls upon a photodetector. The intensity and angular distribution of the scattered radiation is a function of the properties of the scattering particle, notably its size, shape and refractive index.

As with the aperture impedance detector the solution for a particular case is calculated by summing up the contributions of each geometric element. The theory of scattering of electromagnetic radiation has been developed completely (Kerker, 1969) for the particular case of homogeneous spheres (Mie scattering), and computer programs are now available for computing the Mie intensity distribution functions and other relevant quantities. The strong dependence of the angular distribution of scattering on the particle size is illustrated in Figure 2.3. The values of the parameters used in calculating the curves of Figure 2.3 are typical for red blood cells.

Optical system parameters can be chosen so that the measured intensity over a range of angles varies approximately linearly with cell size given that the other factors remain equal. In a typical system using a volume of 90 fl as a calibration point an assumption of strict linearity would yield errors in cell volumes of no more than 12% over the range from 10 fl to 140 fl. The resolution and detection limit of such a system is typically less than 1 fl and is limited by the ratio of the signal voltage to the fluctuations in the dark current of the detector resulting from the detector's resistance. Thus the S/N can be increased linearly with the optical power until the scattered light from the background becomes the limiting noise. Using a high power laser it can approach

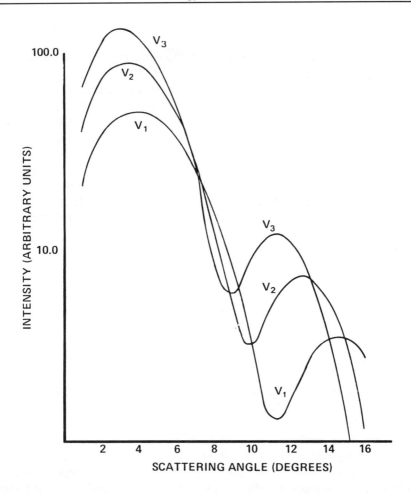

Figure 2.3 Relation between angular distribution of scattering as given by the Mie theory for spherical particles of different size (V_1, V_2, V_3). From Groner (1988). Reprinted by permission of John Wiley & Sons, Inc.

the limit imposed by the light scattering of pure water which is on the order of 0.1 fl.

As with the electrical method practical considerations place restrictions on performance which were not considered in the simple theory. The most important of these is the assumption that all cells have the same relative index of refraction. Since this is not generally true of blood cells a single calibration constant cannot be used for cells of different index of refraction. In addition, unlike the electrical method the optical signals from red blood cells are strictly dependent upon the contents of the cell, not on the integrity of the membrane, therefore resealed red cell ghosts give signals much smaller than those obtained from the original blood cell.

The simple model also assumes that the cells are homogeneous particles. This is a reasonable approximation for RBCs but is a very poor assumption for WBCs, which contain internal structures of varying refractive indices. Thus, the optical method is not suitable for sizing WBCs, and is limited in sizing RBCs due to their variation in shape and hemoglobin content. This problem has been solved for RBCs by isovolumetrically sphering them and comparing the intensity of scatter at different angles. In this case the Mie theory can be used to de-couple the relation between size and index of refraction, yielding two output signals one of which is related to the cell volume and the other to the index of refraction. The second signal can then in turn be related to the cell hemoglobin content.

Detector combinations

The discussions above considered the case in which each cell was detected as a change in the signal from a single detector whose major function was to count cells and determine their size. However, it is possible to obtain from the passage of one cell, two or more signals derived from detectors which are either coincident or adjacent. Figure 2.4 shows an optical detection system in which the beam after striking blood cells contained in a flow cell is divided and sent to two different detectors. One detector is sensitive to the light which was scattered by the cell and the other sensitive to the light which was absorbed by the cell. Thus, information regarding both size and color can be obtained simultaneously. Another example is the case mentioned above where the intensities of laser light scattered at two different angles are compared to eliminate the effects of index of refraction and obtain an accurate size for RBC.

In a similar manner two signals can be obtained simultaneously in the electrical method by superimposing an RF current on the DC aperture current and observing the current changes made by the passage of a cell at both the relatively low frequency and at the RF frequency. In this way two signals, one principally affected by cell size, and one principally affected by cell structure, can be compared.

For a final example consider Figure 2.5 in which the blood cells are passed sequentially through an electrical detector and an optical detector. In this case the sensing volume is defined by both sensors and coincidence may be made more likely. However, provided the two detectors are close together the signals from each cell can be combined and the attributes of the optical method added to those of the electrical method. Obviously, each of the sensors can in turn be combined and the signals

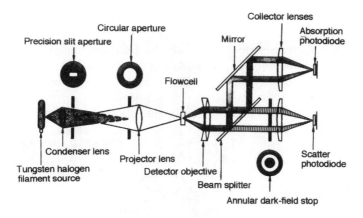

Figure 2.4 Optical detection system with two detectors

multiplied by following the examples presented above for optical and electrical detection methods.

FLUID TRANSPORT TECHNOLOGY

There are three essential elements of the fluid transport technology used in cell counters: the means by which the blood specimen is sampled, the means by which the sample is diluted and processed as well as the means by which the diluted and prepared sample is presented to the cell counting detection station. In the following paragraphs we will discuss the general considerations involved in each of these processes.

Sampling

The principal specimen for analysis in the routine hematology laboratory is venous blood drawn into an anticoagulant containing tube. The type of anticoagulant and the nature of the collection (evacuated container or syringe) are both parameters that can affect the final result and must each be considered either in the design or calibration of the cell counting system. The most commonly used collection method in modern laboratories is a tube which contains liquid ETDA and has been previously evacuated to facilitate the drawing of venous blood.

Although some laboratories still present samples manually to the analyzer there is a growing use of automated samplers in the hematology laboratory worldwide. The basic functions of automated samplers are to store the samples and automatically present them to the instru-

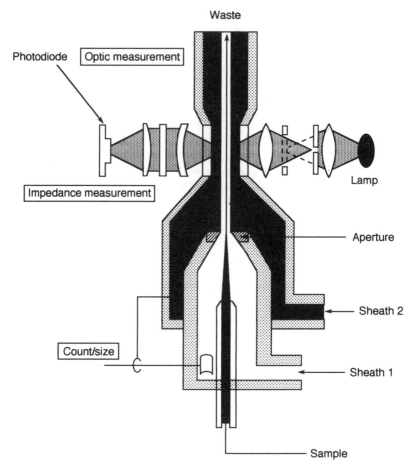

Figure 2.5   System combining an electrical detector and an optical detector
(Roche Diagnostics, Brancheburg, NJ, USA)

ment's sample aspiration station. Typically the sample is identified by a
bar-coded label which is read by the instrument either just before or at
the time of sampling. In these functions hematology samplers are
similar to automated samplers used in automated serum chemistry
testing instruments. There is, however, an important distinction
between the samplers used for automated serum analysis and those
used for hematology. This difference stems from the fact that blood is a
two phase fluid and this is relevant to the fundamental issue of volume
accounting. In order to prevent settling of cells from affecting the
results, the hematology sampler must mix the sample before aspiration.
In early designs of automated samplers for cell counters, mixing was

invasive with a stirrer inserted in the sample and rotated for a period before aspiration. However, this technology was unsatisfactory due to contamination of the sample by material on the stirrer and has largely been replaced. Current hematology samplers either use noninvasive mixing (rotating or rocking the sample container) or mix invasively with the same tube used for aspiration.

In analogy with automated serum chemistry instruments, early automated hematology samplers used a common reservoir or sample cup into which the blood sample was transferred manually from the collection tube. This also proved unsatisfactory for a number of reasons. First, it was not economic. Second, because of the non-Newtonian nature of the blood, it is difficult to pour off an aliquot of specimen without losing volume accounting. Finally, and more important, there was concern regarding personnel safety. This is especially significant in the hematology laboratory where it has been shown that the necessary function of mixing can create aerosols and hence transport bloodborne pathogens. Consequently, most of the modern multiparameter systems feature the ability to sample directly from one or more closed sample collection tubes.

Sample division/dilution processing

Modern hematology analyzers typically divide the original specimen into two or more aliquots which are then diluted and processed in parallel channels prior to counting. The principal concern in dividing and diluting the sample is volume accounting. A well characterized and precise amount of sample fluid must be extracted without affecting the homogeneity of the cells in suspension and then diluted by factors of several hundred to one. The second concern is the volume itself, since the lower the total specimen volume required, the more universally useful is the cell counter. Modern instruments operate on a total of less than 100 microliters of whole blood which is then divided and diluted with a precision of approximately 1%. Thus, the variability in dividing and dispensing the specimen must be less than 1 microliter. In order to achieve this level of precision each successive sample must be loaded without distortion into the same well defined (nondistensible) volume and then dispensed into a larger container together with a diluent. The most commonly used technology for diluting and dispensing of the whole blood sample is a multiport shear valve following the general design of the blood sampling valve introduced by Coulter in the Model S system. In this device, illustrated in Figure 2.6, blood is drawn through and caused to fill one or more small chambers contained within the movable element of the valve. This sample is then captured by the valve movement. Valves of this general design may be made of

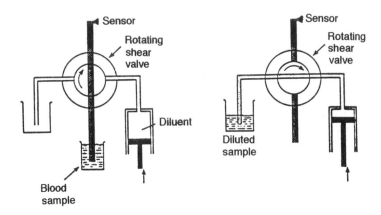

Figure 2.6 An automated dilution method in which diluted blood is aspirated (left) into a capillary chamber contained within a rotating shear valve. After rotation of the valve, the captured sample is forced out (right) by the diluent. From Groner (1988), reprinted by permission of John Wiley & Sons, Inc.

steel or ceramic. The valve is then rotated to isolate these sections by the "shearing action" of the valve face. This same motion connects the isolated sections to their respective diluents. A metered amount of each diluent is then forced through, diluting the sample and depositing the mixture in an incubation or reaction chamber. Depending on the nature of the process, one or more additional reagents may then be added to the incubation/reaction chamber. Thus, a hematology analyzer may be characterized by the number and volume of aliquots taken from the original blood specimen, the dilution factor for each channel and a description of the further processing required for each channel to prepare the sample for counting. In Table 2.1 the sample characteristics are given for some of the modern instruments.

Additional sample processing steps after dividing the sample are designed to enhance the characteristics of the cells which will subsequently be detected in the cell counter and eliminate potential interference. Typically, separate channels are used for determining the total hemoglobin, counting RBCs and platelets, and one or more channels to accomplish the WBC differential.

In the hemoglobin channel red cells are lysed and the hemoglobin converted to a stable form such as methemoglobin or cyanmethemoglobin. The end point is then read with a spectrophotometer. The principal source of error in the determination of hemoglobin is turbidity resulting either from RBC stroma or WBC.

The red blood cells and platelets are typically processed and counted

Table 2.1 Sampling comparison

Systems		Specimen volumes/channel				
		HGB	RBC	WBC 1	WBC 2	WBC 3
Coulter	MAXM/STKS	28 μl	1.6 μl	31 μl	N/A	N/A
Coulter	STKR	28 μl	1.6 μl	N/A	N/A	N/A
TOA	NE-8000	6 μl	4 μl	12 μl	12 μl	12 μl
Technicon	H* (ALL)	2 μl	2 μl	20 μl	20 μl	N/A
Abbott	CD-3500	20 μl	0.6 μl	32 μl	N/A	N/A
Roche	HELIOS/ARGOS 5 part	25 μl	SHARE Hb	25 μl	15 μl	N/A
Roche	HELIOS/ARGOS L.M.G.	25 μl	Share Hb	N/A	N/A	N/A

together using signal size as the principal discriminator between the two cell types. The principal sources of error in this determination are coincidence, discrimination between platelets and spurious noise, and discrimination between large platelets and small red blood cells. Thus, the sample processing for this cell counting channel typically involves a substantial dilution (magnitude determined by the cell counter sensing volume) in a diluent of isotonic saline at a pH of 7.4. In systems where the subsequent cell counter is sensitive to the spherical volume of the red blood cells (see detection methods) detergent and fixative may be added to the diluent to isovolumetrically sphere (Ponder, 1948) and hold the shape of the red blood cells.

The processing of white blood cells is more complex. First, the red blood cells must be eliminated by hemolysis from interfering with the count. Secondly, one or more reagents are used to enhance the discrimination between the cells (see cell identification below). This discrimination is dependent on the technology for cell counting and classification which is generally system specific.

Transport to the detector

In cell counting the cells are counted as the fluid containing them flows past the detection station. The result is a sequence of electrical pulses whose rate is related to the cell concentration x as:

$$r = kxe^{Kx} \tag{1}$$

Where:

r is the rate of pulse arrival (pulses/second),

k is the flow rate in meters/second,

K is the volume of the sensing element in meters cubed.

The exponential factor (Kx) represents explicitly the probability of coincidence (two particles in the sensing zone at the same time). Noting that as an approximation for small values of Kx the exponential may be expanded as:

$$e^{Kx} = 1 + Kx + (Kx)^2 + \ldots$$

we note that for small values of Kx:

$$r = kx$$

thus, as long as the flow rate is constant and sensing volume is small compared to the space between cells, r is a linear function of x. In other words, the count rate is proportional to the cell concentration.

The cell count is then determined either directly through the above relationship by counting for a known time or alternatively by accumulating the total number of cells counted while a known volume of fluid is caused to flow past the detector. In either case the technical problems are to ensure that the flow rate is known and constant during the counting period, that there is no recirculation causing multiple counts for a single cell, and that each cell is detected.

The flow rate is generally controlled by the displacement of a tightly fitting piston or an advancing column of mercury moving in a cylinder of known dimensions. However, the flow geometry is dependent upon the dimensions of the detection system. Figure 2.7 shows two typical

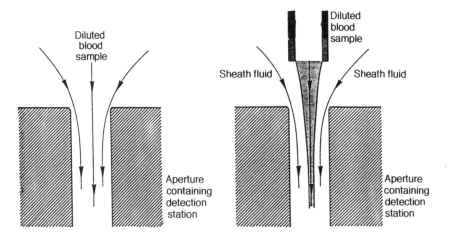

Figure 2.7 Two typical flow cell geometries: (left) cells in suspension are forced through aperture, (right) cells in suspension are injected in a laminar flow system and carried without mixing by a sheath fluid. From Groner (1988), reprinted by permission of John Wiley & Sons, Inc.

flow geometries commonly in use. In the first example the diluted sample fills the aperture containing the detection station. In the other the diluted sample is constrained to the center of the aperture by surrounding it within an inert particle-free sheath fluid.

In the first example, since there is substantial deceleration of the flow at the exit of the aperture, there is a possibility of "swirling" which could create a secondary signal as the particle re-entered or partially re-entered the detection zone. In order to avoid this problem a net fluid flow in the lateral direction is sometimes used to direct the particles as they exit the aperture. This is called the "back swept aperture". Another solution to the problem which was invented by Von Behrens imposes a deflection plate with a hole in it behind the sensing aperture to direct the exiting particles. Figure 2.8 illustrates the operation of the Von Behrens plate.

In the second example, which is generally called hydrodynamic focusing or "sheath flow", the problem of nonaxial particles and recirculation are resolved by constraining the sample flow to the center of the sensing zone. This advantage is gained, however, at the expense of complexity (additional fluid) and the mechanical decoupling of the sample flow rate from the total flow.

These different means of fluid transport are equally applicable to any of the detection methods described above. The important difference between the optical and electrical methods is that regardless of whether a sheath stream is used, the detection volume for the electrical method is determined by the mechanical dimensions of the aperture

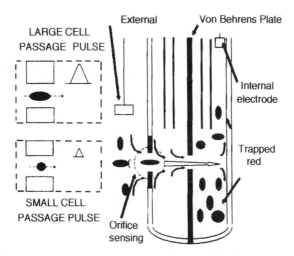

Figure 2.8 Von Behrens plate (courtesy of Abbott Diagnostics, Abbott Park, IL, USA)

while the detection volume of the optical method is determined by the dimensions of the light beam. Thus, by focusing the light in the case of hydrodynamic focusing the sensing volume can be reduced to the size of the sample stream.

SIGNAL PROCESSING

For automated cell counters the output from the detection station is a randomly timed train of electrical signals representing the passage of blood cells. This signal train must be processed in order to create the final result. Processing typically includes:

1. Discrimination, i.e. separating and classifying signals
2. Coincidence correction, i.e. eliminating coincidence error.
3. Results formatting, i.e. organizing the result for use in the laboratory.

The following paragraphs will describe each of these functions in general terms, pointing out the different approaches which may be used.

Discriminating techniques

Cell counting instruments rely on the ability to discriminate on the basis of amplitude the signals of a particular cell class from spurious noise on the one hand, and other cell classes on the other. Three different techniques are in common use in amplitude discrimination between cell signals and spurious noise or other cell types:

1. A-priori thresholding (pre-gating).
2. A-posteriori thresholding (back gating).
3. Curve fitting.

A-priori thresholding (Pre-Gating)
In a-priori thresholding a comparison voltage (threshold) is preset above the noise level in the signal-detection electronic circuit and the cell count derived by counting the number of times the signal level crosses the threshold voltage during the counting period (Figure 2.9). In a-priori thesholding false counts may be registered by noise pulses exceeding the preset threshold, while cells whose signals are lower than the threshold are missed.

A-aposteriori thresholding (Back-Gating)
In a-posteriori thresholding a similar circuit is used to precondition the analog signal. However, with this technique the lower threshold is deliberately set to include some but not all noise pulses. The peak

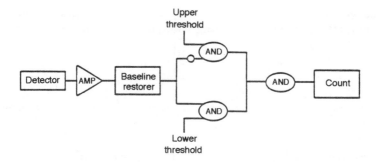

Figure 2.9 Schematic diagram of a detection circuit for a cell counter. From Groner (1988), reprinted by permission of John Wiley & Sons, Inc.

amplitude of each pulse occurring during the counting period is then digitized and the result stored as a histogram of cell number vs signal. This histogram is then analyzed after completion of the counting period. Discrimination thresholds are then set in valleys to isolate regions of the histogram and the cell counts within each region summed up to obtain the cell count. Figure 2.10 (a, b, c) demonstrates the steps in a-posteriori thresholding.

In a-posteriori thresholding by carefully setting the discriminator at the minimum of the histogram the probability of noise exceeding the discriminator is balanced by the probability of the loss of cell count.

Curve fitting
The curve fitting technique is an alternative a-posteriori scheme except instead of simply setting a discrimination threshold the histogram data is subjected to a statistical curve fitting algorithm. The cell count is then obtained by integrating the fitted curve (Figure 2.10d). In this technique the effects of false counts are minimized by the extrapolation of the fitted curve. However, another source of error is introduced through the fitting. If the fit is "not good" the integrated curve will not accurately represent the cell count.

Coincidence correction

The finite volume of the detection station introduces nonlinearity in the relationship between pulse count and cell count, indicated by the exponential factor Kx in the equation (1) above. This is the relationship between the average volume per cell and the volume of the detection station. Although cell counting detectors have relatively small sensing volumes, it is sometimes necessary to apply a correction for the possibi-

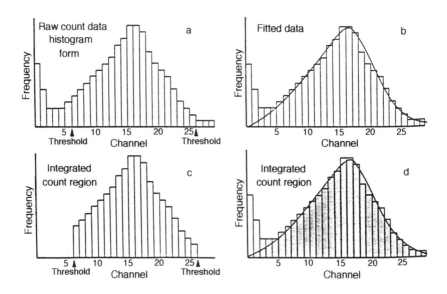

Figure 2.10 A-posteriori thresholding. From Groner (1988), reprinted by permission of John Wiley & Sons, Inc.

lity that more than one cell is in the detection station at the same time, especially when counting red blood cells. This is called coincidence correction. When the sensing volume is well known, coincidence correction can generally be applied effectively using relatively straightforward approaches.

As an example Figure 2.11 shows the geometry for cell counting using optical detection and a sheath flow hydraulic design. For this case since the detection volume has a constant cross section it can also be expressed in terms of the pulse duration that is, the larger the volume the longer it takes to traverse it. Thus, the probability of coincidence is also given by the cell rate times the pulse width or the total time that the sensing volume is occupied. This is called the "dead time". This fact can be used to correct the count:

$$Corrected\ count\ rate = \frac{r}{1 - DT}$$

where:

r is the observed rate,
DT is the dead time.

Although coincidence correction is generally quite effective, a problem in coincidence correction arises when more than one cell type is being

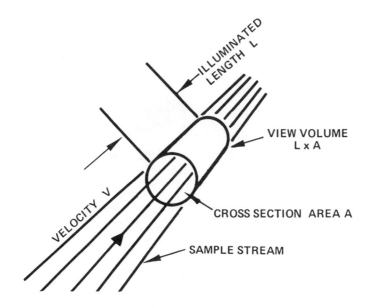

Figure 2.11 Typical geometry of cell counting using optical detection and a sheath flow hydraulic design. From Groner (1988), reprinted by permission of John Wiley & Sons, Inc.

enumerated by the same detector, as when red cells and platelets are counted at the same dilution. When cells of different types are in coincidence, one type is usually favored by the classification process and hence the coincidence correction must be different for each. The proper corrections are determined by calculating the probability of detection for each cell type specifically. This involves calculating the additional probabilities of coincidence (e.g. type a with a, a with b, b with b) and convolving with the bias of the classification process for cross-type events.

CELL SIZING

A principal feature of the modern hematology analyzers is the ability to measure cell size in addition to counting the cells by class and then report information regarding the size and size distribution of the cells. The technology questions appear straightforward: first, can a precise relationship between signal size and cell size be etablished and maintained; second, can a standard information format be applied so that results can be presented for diagnostic analysis? However, there are additional issues which are much more complex.

One issue involves the relationship between cell size as an in-vitro

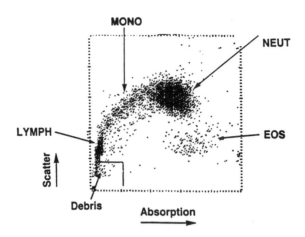

Figure 2.12 A cytogram or scatterplot. Each dot represents the amplitude of two optical measurements made on a single cell. EOS, eosinophils; LYMPH, lymphocytes; MONO, monocytes; NEUT, neutrophils. From Groner (1988), reprinted by permission of John Wiley & Sons, Inc.

parameter and cell size as an in-vivo parameter. The shape and size of blood cells are not well characterized constants since living cells can and do change both their size and shape in vivo. Further, the action of anticoagulant, in-vitro storage conditions and the diluting fluid can and will modify both the size and shapes of cells in vitro. Thus, even accurate results obtained on an in-vitro blood sample concerning the size or distribution of size are not immediately interpretable since they may as easily reflect an in-vitro storage condition as an in-vitro diagnostic one.

The first practical application of cell sizing was the determination of the mean red blood cell volume, which eliminated the need to centrifuge and pack the cells in order to obtain the red cell indices. More recently data about the size distribution of RBCs (RDW) and platelets (MPV) have been incorporated in the routine "blood count". In addition, size discrimination has been used effectively as an aid to the classification of leukocytes.

In the section on detection we have seen how a signal proportional to size can be obtained from either optical or aperture impedance detectors. In the case of the optical detection of particles larger than the wavelength of light (most cells) shape is a principal interference and must be known and controlled typically by sphering the cells. In the electrical method the principal source of error is the variation in signal resulting from nonaxial cell trajectories. For accurate sizing these must be controlled by hydrodynamic focusing (sheath stream flow cell) or eliminated by pulse editing. Shape is also a factor in sizing with the electrical method, but provided it is controlled or well described the error can be eliminated by a calibration factor.

Sizing by means of optical or aperture impedance methods is also sensitive to changes in the physical properties of the particles. For instance, if the red cells were partially hemolyzed, without a change in red cell volume, the volume isolated inside the red cell membrane would not be affected; hence, the size as seen by the electrical method would remain constant. The index of refraction would be altered dramatically because of loss of hemoglobin and as a result the intensity of scattered light would change. Unless the optical detection system was able to separate changes in the size of the sphere from changes in its index of refraction, a difference between methods would result.

For relatively simple particles, such as well characterized dielectric spheres such as red cells, particle size can be measured with either method of detection once interferences are known and corrected for. After applying calibration factors to eliminate bias, a good correlation can be obtained between them. Figure 2.13 shows the results obtained for sizing the RBCs from various mammalian species when the methods are compared. In this experiment care was taken to eliminate factors such as shape which would interfere with the correlation between measurements.

As we move away from relatively simple particles like RBCs the potential for differences between the methods becomes greater. Changes in shape or internal constitution of the particles will affect both systems, but in a completely uncorrelated manner. Thus agreement in the results obtained by different detection methods for sizing platelets and WBCs cannot be expected to be as good as that for RBCs.

As a result of improvements in cell processing technology, cell counting technology, and also computer technology, it is possible to obtain, in addition to the mean cell volume, information regarding the distribution of sizes of individual cells. Although there is an intuitive feeling that data showing intersample and intrasample variations in cell size distribution must have clinical meaning the interpretations are not yet well established. One part of the problem is that the results from different systems are not equivalent. Another is the problems mentioned above regarding in-vitro vs in-vivo storage changes. Yet a third is the inability to relate the results to the previous observations of microscopic morphology. The diagnostic guideposts which have been achieved over the years relating cell size to disease have been established through microscopic cell morphology on prepared films in which the cells are flattened and dried. In this case the relationship between the observed cell size and the true cell size (in-vitro or in-vivo) is not

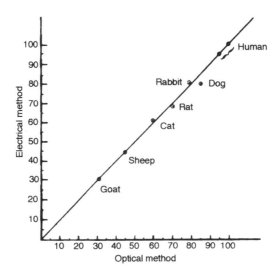

Figure 2.13   Comparison of electrical and optical methods for sizing animal
blood cells

always known. However, it is also possible that the data is just too
ambiguous to be useful.

As an example consider the red cell distribution width which is probably the best understood of the cell size parameters. It is reasonably
stable, can be accurately determined, and is analogous to anisocytosis
as reported by microscopic morphology (England, 1982). Thus, given a
standard for presenting results (ICSH, 1982), a precise quantitation of
the red cell distribution width can be incorporated as part of the
routine hematology results. However, in spite of attempts to interpret it
(Bessman, 1985) there remains doubt that this quantity adds any clear
value to the laboratory results easily translatable in terms of diagnosis
or patient management. Thus, the only real use of the RDW may be as
a flag for the laboratorian to trigger further more specific investigation.

The situation with platelet size parameters is even worse, where in-
vitro changes are dramatic due to changes in size with storage, method
errors are appreciable, and no standardization for reporting results has
been yet accepted.

CELL IDENTIFICATION

Discrimination of cells by class in cell counting generally depends
upon a discrimination within the instrument on the basis of signal
amplitudes. It was stated above that the signal results from the dis-

turbance of an electromagnetic field and hence is influenced by the cell's physical properties. We have seen how cell size and shape can alter the signal amplitude with both aperture impedance and optical detection systems. In addition, other physical properties of the cell can influence the signal when a detector is appropriately tuned to their presence; e.g. the color of the cell will affect the light transmitted by the detection zone at an appropriation absorption wavelength. Thus, a detector tuned to this signal by the use of a color filter can be used to measure the stain uptake of each cell as it is counted. Similarly, a light detector can be tuned to the light emitted (fluorescence) from the cell as it crosses an optical detection zone by a combination of masking and filtering. Such a detector can be used to aid in the discrimination of cells on the basis of their fluorescent properties, either naturally occurring fluorescence or as a result of staining with a fluorescent dye.

In general the technology of cell identification will involve the combination of two elements. The first element is the enhancement of the distinction between classes of cells by emphasizing one or more of the cell's physical properties (size, color, fluorescence, etc.). The second element involves tuning one or more detection stations to that particular physical property through a combination of spatial and spectral filtering (for optical detectors) or frequencies (for electrical detectors). The cell signal may then be processed and the cell classified on the basis of the resulting signal amplitude. In the identification of the WBC sub-classes the principal features used by modern hematology systems are the size and internal structure of the cells. After lysing the RBC, lymphocytes are identified by their size while granulocytes are identified by their internal structure. In some cases the internal constituents may be further enhanced by staining. In general, the trade-off is between the complexity of the methods for modifying the blood cells versus the complexity of the detection technology. That is, when more channels and reagents are used for identification the detectors are less complex. The opposite is also true.

The principal issues involved in the technology for cell identification result from alternative choices in tagging cell types. For example, consider the classifying of monocytes. The monocyte is traditionally distinguished by microscopy in a Wright–Giemsa stained slide as a mononuclear cell which is usually larger than a lymphocyte. It has a grey-blue cytoplasm containing dustlike and/or discrete azurophilic granules. The monocyte has been recognized in cell counting instruments on the basis of its relative size, non-specific esterase activity, and relative peroxidase activity. Further, it has been classified by flow cytometry on the basis of the reaction of surface proteins with certain monoclonal antibodies. Thus, we have five alternative definitions of the monocyte.

These definitions may agree in general; however, there will be many instances in which they disagree leading to ambiguity in the monocyte count.

Even when the definitions of a cell class are similar in two instruments ambiguity can still result from more subtle differences. For example: consider the normal lymphocyte which is defined in traditional microscopy as a relatively small cell with dense chromatin and basophilic cytoplasm. Cell counters universally classify the lymphocyte after lysing the red blood cells on the basis signal size as the smallest leukocyte. However, there is no absolute rule as to how to set the "size" threshold. Therefore, the difference between technology yields perceptible method biases in lymphocyte count (Simson and Groner, 1995), and biases for some lymphocytes can occur even within a single technology as a result of variation in the discrimination algorithm (Cohen *et al.*, 1993).

MULTIPLE CELL CLASSIFICATION

The ultimate task for a cell counter is to enumerate cells accurately within a defined class on the basis of signal characteristics. For the simple cell counter this may be done by merely discriminating signals from spurious noise (see discriminating techniques above), and correcting for coincidence. However, the problems discussed above of coincidence and signal processing become more challenging when the signals must be further characterized and cells counted and classified into more than one category.

For illustration consider the idealized histogram shown in Figure 2.14. In this case two discrete classes of particles, one (Particle A) of signal level 6 and one (Particle B) of signal level 10, must be classified. Although the particle signals are discrete, there is a noise background whose average value is 2. As can be seen, three classes of coincident particles result: one for two particles of each class at 12 and 20; and one for the mixed class at 18. In analogy with the single class coincidence problem the total count rate or dead time can be used to determine how large the loss due to coincidence is. However, it gives no indication of how to apply the correction should the lost counts be added to the concentration of Particle A, Particle B or divided between them. In fact, for this two class coincidence problem the solution is only tractable when the relative concentrations of particles are known; in which case we would not need to count them accurately. Thus, the tradeoffs in approaching the cell classification problem involve the balance of three factors: the number of channels, the dilution, and the residual coincidence error. Obviously if each channel counts a single class the complexity of the two class coincidence problem is avoided, but cost, in terms of

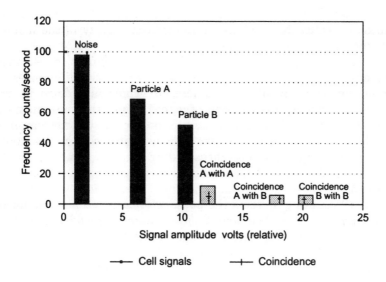

Figure 2.14 Illustration of an idealized two-class coincidence problem (no
biologic variation) as a signal amplitude histogram

both hardware and consumables, is sacrificed. Alternately, even the two
class coincidence error can be mitigated by sufficient dilution. However,
in this case, either counting precision or throughput must be sacrificed.
Modern cell counters use multiple cell classification for erythrocytes and
platelets as well as in the sub-classification of leukocytes. Typically,
dilution is used to mitigate the two class coincidence problem for the
WBC. However, due to the low relative frequency of platelets this is not
possible for a combined RBC and platelet counting channel. In this case,
approximations are generally used based on assumptions regarding the
relative numbers of cells (Groner and Epstein, 1982).

RESULTS FORMATTING

The results of measurements performed with cell counting instruments
may be reported to the laboratory in one or more of three different techniques: numerical counts, histograms and cytograms. The following
paragraphs will briefly describe and define each of these different
formats.

Numerical results
In this format the results of the measurements performed with the cell
counting instruments are presented by a simple number representing

the cell concentration in number per unit volume. Occasionally, such as in sub-classification of WBC, the concentration may also be represented as a percentage of the total class.

Histograms
In this format the results are displayed graphically, illustrating by means of a frequency distribution of signal height the concentration of cells as a function of the signal amplitude (or the distribution of cell size). The histogram technique was demonstrated in Figure 2.10 as an illustration of one dimensional thresholding.

Cytograms
In some cell counting systems the passage of each cell may be noted by two detectors as described above. For example, consider the case in counting with an optical method when one detector is used to measure the light scattered by each cell and another detector used to measure the light absorbed. The two signal amplitude which results can be plotted in a graphic form by representing each cell as a point in a graph whose distance from the origin is represented by the signal amplitude in each of the two detection channels. This form of graphic display may be called a cytogram. Figure 2.12 demonstrates the cytogram which is produced by measuring the scatter and absorption of white blood cells after they have been treated with a special enzyme stain.

REFERENCES

Bessman, J.D. (1985) More on the RDW [letter]. *Am. J. Clin. Pathol.* **84**(6): 773.

Cohen, A.J., Peerschke, E. and Stegbegel, R.T. (1993) A comparison of the Coulter STKS, Coulter S +IV and manual analysis of white blood cell differential counts in human immunodeficiency virus infected population. *Amer. J. Clin. Pathol.* **100**: 611.

Coulter, W.H. (1956) High speed automatic blood cell counter and cell size analyzer. *Proceedings of the National Electronics Conference* **12**: 1034–40.

England, J.M. (1982) The analysis and interpretation of cell size distribution curves in hematology; a review. In Van Assendelft, O.W. and England, J.M. (eds.) *Advances in Hematological Methods: The Blood Count*, pp. 109–124. CRC Press, Boca Raton.

Goldsmith, H.L. and Karino, T. (1980) Physical and mathematical models of blood flow. In *Erythrocyte Mechanics and Blood Flow*, Volume 13. Kroc foundation Series. Alan R. Liss, NY.

Groner, W. (1988) Cell counters. In Webster, J. (ed.) *Encyclopedia of Medical Devices*. J. Wiley, New York.

Groner, W. and Epstein, E. (1982) Counting and sizing of blood cells using light scattering. In van Assendelft, O.W. and England, J.M. (eds.) *Advances in Hematological Methods: the Blood Count*, pp. 73–84. CRC Press, Boca Raton.

ICSH (1982) Recommendations for the analysis of red cell, white cell and platelet size distribution curves. I. General Principles. *J. Clin. Pathol.* **35**: 1320–2.

Kerker, M. (1969) *The scattering of Light and Other Electromagnetic Radiation.* Academic Press, NY.

Kubitschek, H.E. (1960) Electronic measurement of particle size. *Res. Appl. Ind.* **13**: 128.

Ponder, E. (1948) *Hemolysis and Related Phenomena.* Grune & Stratton, NY.

Simson, E. and Groner, W. (1995) Variability in absolute lymphocyte counts obtained by automated cell counters. *Cytometry* **22**: 26–34.

Tycko, D.H., Metz, M.H., Epstein, E.A. and Grinbaum, A. (1985) Flowcytometric light scattering measurement of red blood cell volume and hemoglobin concentration. *Appl. Opt.* **24**: 1355.

FURTHER READING

Bessis, M. (1973) *Living Blood Cells and Their Ultrastructure.* Springer-Verlag, Berlin and New York.

Bull, B.S. (1967) A semiautomatic micro sample dilutor. *Am. J. Clin. Pathol.* **47**: 545.

Coulter, W.H. (1962) *Instruction Manual to the Coulter Counter Model B.*

Crosland Taylor, P.J. (1953) A device for counting small particles suspended in a fluid through a tube. *Nature (London)* **171**: 37.

Crosland Taylor, P.J., Stewart, J.W. and Haggis, G. (1958) An electronic blood counting machine. *Blood* **13**: 398–409.

England, J.M. (1985) Future needs and expected trends in peripheral blood cell analysis: erythrocyte histograms. *Blood Cells.* **11**(1): 61–76.

Freeman, M.F. and Tukey, J.W. (1950) Transformation related to the angular and square root. *Ann. Math. Stat.* **21**: 607.

Fricke, H. (1953) Relation of permittivity of biological cell suspensions to fractional cell volume. *Nature* **172**: 731–2.

Koepke, J. (ed.), (1984) *Laboratory Hematology*, Churchill-Livingstone, Edinburgh and London.

Lewis, S.M. (1970) Pipettes and pipetting in haemoglobinometry. In Astaldi, G., Sirtoni, C. and Vanzette, G. (eds.) *Standardization in Hematology*, p. 45. Franco Angeli, Milan.

Rideout, J.M., Renshaw, A. and Snook, M. (1978) Swizzlestick-Novel positive displacement microliter diluting device. *Anal. Biochem.* **19**: 747.

Roberts, F. and Young, J.Z. (1952) A flying-spot microscope. *Nature (London)* **169**: 518.

Wintrobe, M.M. (1981) *Clinical Hematology*, 8th edn, pp. 1–26. Lea & Febiger, Philadelphia, PA.

Chapter 3

Description of Modern Systems

INTRODUCTION AND OVERVIEW OF CURRENT PRODUCTS

In this chapter we will discuss the currently available commercial systems that automatically produce a complete blood count including at least five sub-classes of WBC. These modern hematology analyzers are highly developed and use sophisticated technology to integrate their operation into routine laboratories. Blood specimens in their collection containers may be introduced directly into the sampling system. The analyzers automatically read bar-code labels and interface with the Laboratory Information System for down-loading test requests and demographics as well as returning results. Specimen processing rates of greater than 100 samples per hour can be obtained. In addition, each of the systems has various customer selected options covering a wide range of internal computer capability that allow: setting of flags, storing quality control (QC) results, and producing graphic reports on specimens and QC materials.

In the following discussions the focus will be primarily on the technical aspects of these modern hematology analyzers. We will detail what these systems do and what technology is used by describing the methods used by each manufacturer. We will then summarize by comparing the methods and technology for each determination across the various systems. First we will briefly review the product line for each manufacturer.

There are currently five manufacturers marketing automated cell counting systems which perform (in addition to the traditional automated CBC) a "complete leukocyte differential", additional cell size parameters, and flagging for abnormal specimens.

1. Coulter Corporation, Miami, Florida 33116, USA
2. TOA Medical Electronics Co., Ltd, Kobe, Japan

Practical Guide to Modern Hematology Analyzers. W. Groner and E. Simson
© 1995 John Wiley & Sons Ltd

3. Bayer Diagnostics, Tarrytown, New York 10591, USA
4. Abbott Diagnostic Division, Abbott Park, IL 60064, USA
5. Roche Diagnostic Systems, Brancheburg, New Jersey 08876, USA

Coulter

The Coulter Corporation, which was formed by the inventor of aperture impedance cell counting, manufactures and distributes a wide range of cell counters for research, industrial and medical use. Of particular interest to the current discussion are two systems which provide a CBC plus full WBC differential, the Coulter MAXM shown in Plate I and the Coulter STKS shown in Figure 3.1. These two systems use identical methods to produce a completely automated 20 parameter output including the traditional eight parameter CBC, both percentage and absolute counts for each of five classes of white blood cells and two cell size parameters. An automated reticulocyte count is also possible on these systems after an off-line specimen preparation. Coulter also manufactures the ONYX shown in Figure 3.2 and the MD16 shown in Figure 3.3 which automatically count and report 16 parameters subclassifying the WBC into three groups: lymphocytes, granulocytes and mononuclear cells.

TOA (Sysmex)

TOA Medical Electronics also manufactures and distributes worldwide a broad line of cell counters. These instruments are distributed in

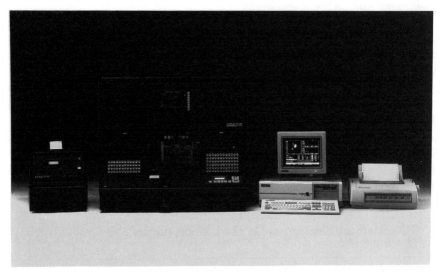

Figure 3.1 The Coulter STKS (Coulter Corporation, Hialeah, FL, USA)

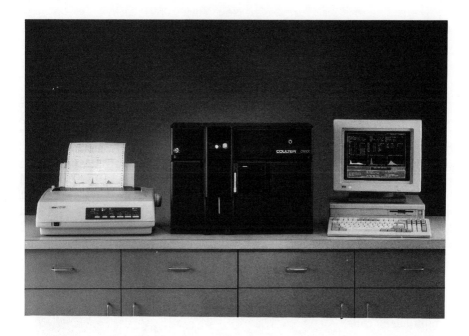

Figure 3.2 The Coulter ONYX (Coulter Corporation, Hialeah, FL, USA)

North America and Europe by the Sysmex Corp. Of particular interest is the NE-8000 and the SE-9000 shown in Plate II. These systems automatically process whole blood specimens and produce a 23 parameter output including: the traditional eight parameter CBC, complete classification of both percentage and absolute counts for the five mature white blood cell classes, and five cell size parameters. The TOA Corp. also manufactures a smaller system, the NE-1500 shown in Figure 3.4. The TOA Corp. has recently introduced into the hematology laboratory the concept of coupling work stations along a specimen transport track such as the HS system shown in Figure 3.5. The HS (Hematology System) and the NE-alpha and the SE-alpha are complete work stations mechanically coupling the NE-8000 with a slide preparation unit that makes blood films. Additional NE-8000 (s), and an automated reticulocyte counter the R-3000, can be connected to the HS.

Bayer Diagnostic

Bayer Diagnostic manufactures and distributes worldwide a broad line of highly automated instruments for the clinical laboratory, including

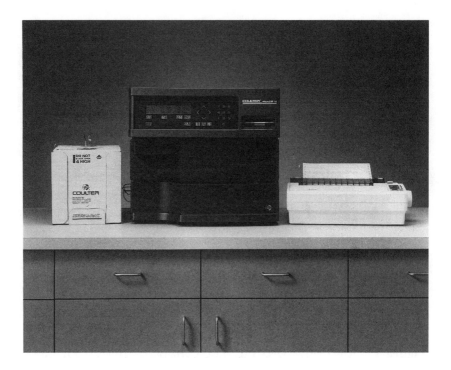

Figure 3.3   The Coulter MD16 (Coulter Corporation, Hialeah, FL, USA)

the line of cell counters under the Technicon trade mark. Each of the counters produces an automated result consisting of 25 parameters and including: the traditional eight parameter CBC, both absolute and per-centage counts for each of six WBC sub-classes and five cell size para-meters. The Bayer line consists of the Technicon H*1 shown in Figure 3.6 which is a smaller system, the larger Technicon H*2 shown in Figure 3.7 and the Technicon H*3 shown in Plate III. A reticulocyte count is available with the H*3 after an off-line preparation step. The H*3 is available in two sizes, the H*3RTX at 102 samples per hour and the H*3RTC at 60 samples per hour.

Abbott Diagnostics

The Abbott Corp. also manufactures and distributes worldwide a broad line of instruments for the diagnostic laboratory including a complete line of hematology analyzers marketed under the Cell-Dyn trade name. These include two multiparameter cell counters (the Cell-Dyn 3000 and

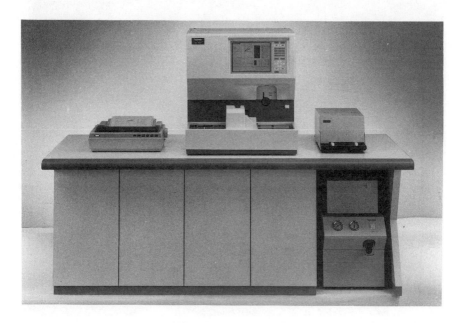

Figure 3.4 The TOA NE-1500 (Sysmex Corporation, Long Grove, IL, USA)

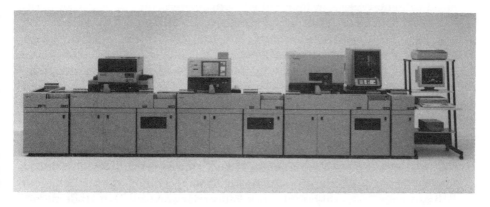

Figure 3.5 The TOA HS (Sysmex Corporation, Long Grove, IL, USA)

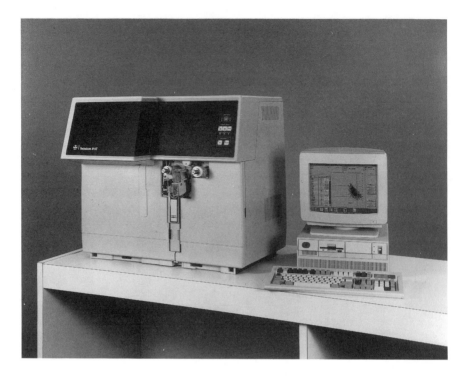

Figure 3.6 The Technicon H*1 (Bayer Diagnostics, Tarrytown, NY, USA)

the more recently introduced Cell-Dyn 3500 shown in Plate IV) which produces a 22 parameter result including: an eight parameter CBC, both percentage and absolute counts of each of the five mature white blood cell sub-types and four cell size parameters.

The Abbott Corp. also distributes smaller cell counters such as the Cell-Dyn 1700 (shown in Figure 3.8) and the Cell-Dyn 1600. These systems produce an 18 parameter output including an eight parameter CBC, six WBC differential parameters and four cell size parameters.

Roche Diagnostic systems

The Roche Corp. also produces and distributes a broad line of diagnostic instruments including a series of cell counters originally introduced under the trade name ABX. These include the fully automated COBAS ARGOS shown in Plate V and the expandable COBAS HELIOS shown in Figure 3.9. Each of these systems is available in two optional config-

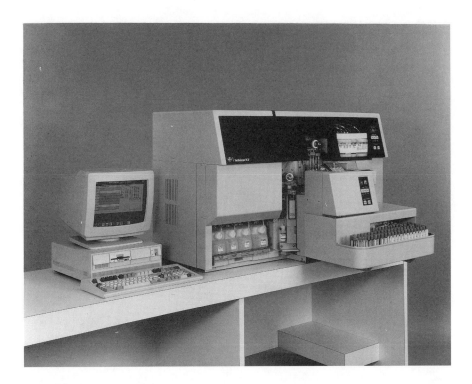

Figure 3.7 The Technicon H*2 (Bayer Diagnostics, Tarrytown, NY, USA)

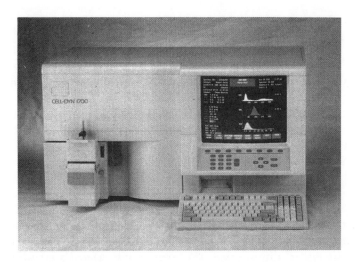

Figure 3.8 The Cell-Dyn 1700 (Abbott Diagnostics, Abbott Park, IL, USA)

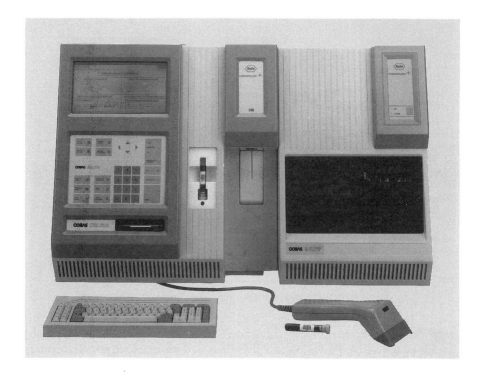

Figure 3.9 The COBAS HELIOS (Roche Diagnostics, Brancheburg, NJ, USA)

urations; one of the options includes a 26 parameter output consisting of an eight parameter CBC seven part WBC differential and five cell size parameters. The other option is with a 20 parameter output consisting of an eight parameter CBC, a limited three part WBC differential, two WBC flags and five cell size parameters. Roche also distributes a smaller system, the COBAS MINOS which produces a 16 parameter CBC including only an eight parameter CBC, three sub-classes of leukocyte and two cell size parameters.

Table 3.1 summarizes the measurement parameters available on each of the multiparameter cell counters mentioned above in general categories. In addition, to the well established eight parameter CBC and the five part differential (10 parameters) there are various new parameters some of which are system specific.

Table 3.1 Summary of commercial systems in terms of output system parameters

Manufacturer	System	Standard CBC (8)	Partial diff. (6)	Full diff. (10)	RBC size	Platelet size	Total
Coulter	STKS	√		√	1	1	20
Coulter	STKR	√	√		1	1	16
Coulter	MAXM	√		√	1	1	20
Coulter	ONYX	√	√		1	1	16
Coulter	MD-16	√	√		1	1	16
TOA	NE-8000	√		√	2	3	23
TOA	SE-9000	√		√	2	3	23
TOA	NE-1500	√		√	2	1	21
Bayer	H*1	√		12*	2	3	25
Bayer	H*2	√		12*	2	3	25
Bayer	H*3	√		12*	2	3	25
Abbott	CD-3500	√		√	1	3	22
Abbott	CD-1700	√	6		1	3	18
Roche	ARGOS 5	√		14*	1	3	26
Roche	HELIOS 5	√		14*	1	3	26
Roche	ARGOS/ HELIOS LMG	√	8*		1	3	20
Roche	MINOS	√	√		1	1	16

*Additional cell classifications not directly relatable to the reference visual differential.

SYSTEM DESCRIPTIONS

In describing the methods used in the commercial systems we will organize the discussion in terms of common functional elements. Figure 3.10 shows a simplified functional block diagram of a multiparameter cell counter. It does not represent any particular instrument, but attempts to illustrate the common steps by which a specimen of anticoagulated whole blood is transformed into a series of analytic results to be used for diagnostic purposes. In the first step (sampling) the blood specimen is aspirated and divided into samples for two or more parallel sample processing channels. In the second step (sample processing methods) the blood specimens are diluted and treated in a manner which will facilitate the counting or measurement of the cells of interest. It is in this step that cell staining and/or differential lysis is employed to distinguish the cells of interest. In the third step the measurements (typically cell count and size) are made on each sample and stored as electrical signals. In the final step (signal processing) the electrical signals are conditioned by system specific algorithms into a set of

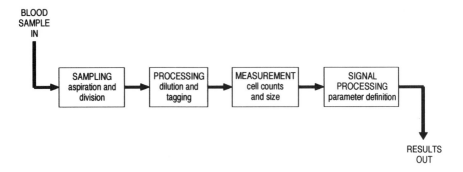

Figure 3.10   Simplified functional block diagram of a multiparameter cell
counting system

reported results including cell counts, indices, and abnormal flags.
Another way of thinking of this step is as "parameter definition" since
in this step the algorithms define the reported parameters.

In the following sections we will describe these functions by discussing the nature of the technologies used by each manufacturer. We will
attempt to keep track of the issues discussed in the previous chapter
on the fundamentals of cell counting technology and try to point out
how each of the manufacturers has addressed them in their system
design. For convenience in each case we will follow the same route as
the specimen, starting with the automated sampler and ending with
the results.

THE COULTER SYSTEMS

Coulter sampling

The Coulter STKS system, first introduced in 1989, and the MAXM
introduced in 1991, feature an automated, closed tube sampler. The
individual sampler of the Coulter MAXM system extracts the sample
from the sealed specimen collection tube after it has been mixed by the
operator. The MAXM system is also available in an automated
sampling version with 25 specimen capacity. Both the STKS and the
MAXM can sample pre-diluted specimens in an open tube sampling
mode.

In the Coulter STKS automated sampler, specimens in their sealed
collection tubes are loaded in cassettes of 12 each and then "stacked"
(up to 144 specimens) awaiting aspiration. Sample racks are mixed by
rocking for greater than two minutes prior to aspiration.

In all cases the blood specimen is drawn through a blood sampling shear valve containing three isolation chambers. In the first chamber 28-μl of specimen is captured for the WBC count and hemoglobin channel. In a second chamber 1.6 μl are captured for counting of RBC and platelets. A third segment of 31 μl is captured for the WBC differential.

Coulter processing methods

The systems employ up to three automated cell preparation methods. One method is used for hemoglobin, a second method for counting red cells and platelets, and the third method only on those systems providing a "complete differential" for determining the white cell differential. In all Coulter systems an independent white cell count is obtained from the hemoglobin method after the determination of hemoglobin. Coulter also offers an off-line method for counting reticulocytes.

The hemoglobin method

In the hemoglobin method whole blood is diluted with a proprietary reagent to a final dilution of 1 part to 251. The action of the reagent is to hemolyze the red cells and convert hemoglobin to a stable form for spectral photometric measurements. White blood cells remain intact and are available for counting and sizing which is accomplished before the determination of hemoglobin. The action of the reagent on the WBC enhances the size difference between cell types. For those systems with only a partial WBC differential, the WBC differential is also obtained from signal size data obtained from this channel.

RBC and platelets

The RBC/platelet method simply consists of a single step dilution to a final dilution of one part specimen to 6250 parts of a buffered isotonic diluent.

White blood cells differential

In the white blood cell method whole blood is diluted with a single reagent to a final dilution of one part to 50. The action of the reagent is to destroy the red blood cells and platelets while maintaining the white blood cells in their near native state for analysis in the Coulter VCS channel, which measures volume, conductivity and light scatter simultaneously, as described below.

Reticulocytes

Coulter has recently added a method for counting reticulocytes on both the STKS and MAXM systems after an off-line preparation in which the specimens are manually stained and diluted. The percentage of reticulocytes is determined in the VCS channel. The staining method uses new methylene blue to color the RNA.

Coulter measurement technology

The measurement technology consists of a hemoglobin colorimeter centred at 525 nm and three cell counters. Two of the cell counters are based on DC aperture impedance while the third employs the multiple transducer VCS technology, combining measurements of DC aperture impedance (V), RF aperture impedance and light scatter (S).

The aperture impedance cell counter

In the aperture impedance counters, vacuum is used to draw samples of the cell suspension (without hydrodynamic focusing) simultaneously through each of three apertures. At the same time, sweep flow is drawn behind the apertures to prevent cells from re-entering the sensing zone. A measurement of the number and volume of cells pulled through each aperture is made and the three results compared for consistency. If all results are consistent, the results are averaged. However, if one aperture has inconsistent results, the data is subject to further analysis and the results from that aperture are voted out. If more than one result is inconsistent the parameter is voted out.

In the aperture impedance cell counters, apertures of 50 μm in diameter and 60 μm in length are used for the RBC/platelet method, while apertures of 100 μm in diameter and 75 μm in length are used for the WBC counting methods. In the Coulter RBC/platelet method, pulse width editing is used to eliminate nonaxial trajectories, and coincidence correction is used to correct the RBC count. In the case of low platelets the time of counting is extended.

The Coulter VCS cell counter

For the WBC differential, Coulter uses a multiparameter sensing system with a triple transducer module. Three measurements are made (volume, conductivity and scatter) as each cell passes through the flow cell. A low frequency (DC) impedance measurement defines the volume while a high frequency conductivity measurement indicates the internal conductivity. A light scattering measurement indicates the structure and shape of each cell. The light scattering measurement is derived from the light scattered by a helium neon laser. Hydrodynamic focusing is used with the Coulter VCS cell counting system. Plate VI shows the cytogram indicating the output of the Coulter VCS cell counter on a normal specimen, when the DC aperture impedance signal is shown as the Y axis and the laser light scatter signal as the X axis.

Coulter parameter definition techniques

In the Coulter systems, the signals obtained for RBCs and platelets are analyzed in the following manner: Platelets and RBCs are discriminated by means of a fixed threshold at a signal equivalent of 37 μm^3. Then the histograms from each set of signals are fitted and the size distribution calculated from the fitted curves. For platelets a log normal distribution is used while a normal distribution is used for red blood cells. Rather than discriminate between platelets and noise, the platelet count is derived from the integral of the platelet fit whenever the fit is good enough. When there is a poor fit the platelet count is obtained by discriminating with a fixed threshold at a signal equivalent of 2 μm^3.

In the VCS analysis a-posteriori discrimination (see Chapter 2) is used in each of the three signal dimensions. As an example, consider the cytogram obtained when the DC aperture impedance signal is plotted as the Y axis and the optical scatter signal as the X axis. Figure 3.11 shows an example of the discrimination of a normal leukocyte specimen in the VCS channel. Note a series of rectangular discriminating thresholds resulting from individual a-posteriori thresholding.

In the white blood cell counting channel a single a-priori threshold is used to isolate leukocytes.

Qualitatively abnormal specimens are flagged for blasts, variant, lymphs and immature granulocytes. These flags are derived on the basis of the analysis of signal distributions in the VCS signal output.

THE TOA (SYSMEX) SYSTEMS

TOA sampling

The Sysmex NE-8000 system, which was introduced in 1989, provides an automated, closed tube sampling system, or alternative manual sampling from an open specimen container.

The automated sampler uses a rack transport system with each rack containing 10 sealed specimen tubes. Racks are available for 75 mm long specimen containers of 12 mm, 13 mm, 14 mm and 15 mm diameter. The tubes are mixed by a robotic arm. Each tube is inverted a total of 10 times before aspiration.

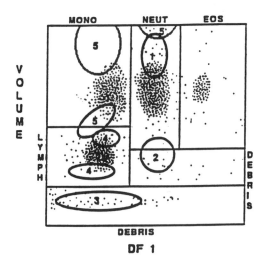

Figure 3.11 Example of the cell classification scheme for the Coulter systems, showing the location of normal and abnormal cells. Y axis, aperture impedance volume; X axis, light scatter. 1, Suspect bands/immature granulocytes; 2, suspect, damaged or aged neutrophils; 3, suspect cellular debris, NRBC, platelet clumps; 4, suspect variant lymphocytes; 5, suspect blasts. MONO, monocytes; NEUT, neutrophils; EOS, eosinophils; LYMPH, lymphocytes. (Coulter Corporation, Hialeah, FL, USA)

The NE-8000 system can also aspirate pre-mixed specimen tubes which are presented manually to the aspiration port. Pre-diluted and mixed capillary specimens can also be aspirated through a separate aspiration station.

In the TOA NE-Series, the specimen is drawn into a sample rotor (shear) valve where five separate samples are isolated. A 6 μl sample is used for the hemoglobin determination, a 4 μl sample is used for the sizing and counting of RBC/platelets, and separate 12 μl segments are used for the WBC count and differential. In the SE-9000, seven separate samples are isolated: 3 μl for hemoglobin, 4 μl for RBC/lose, 2.4 μl for counting WBC, three separate segments for the WBC differential and 2.4 μl for immaturity evaluation and flagging.

TOA processing methods

Up to five separate automated methods are employed in the hematology analyzers, the first for the determination of hemoglobin, the second for counting and sizing of RBC/ platelet, and three separate methods for sub-classifications of white blood cells. A separate instrument is used for performing an automated reticulocyte count.

Hemoglobin

The hemoglobin method uses a rapid transformation of hemoglobin into a stable form by the action of a surfactant lysing agent (sodium laurel sulfate) which is accomplished in less than 40 seconds. The product is a stable complex of the sodium laurel sulfate (SLS) with methemoglobin which has a broad absorption peak at 550 nm. Whole blood is first diluted 1:333 with a diluent. 0.500 ml of the lysing reagent is then added to obtain a final dilution of 1 part to 500. The method does not use cyanide to eliminate problems of waste disposal.

RBC and platelets

In the RBC/platelet method, whole blood is simply diluted to a final dilution of 500 to 1 in an isotonic saline diluent.

WBC

The WBC method: used on the NE-8000 also distinguishes three populations: lymphocytes, monocytes and granulocytes. In this method, whole blood is diluted in two steps into reagents containing formaldehyde and a lysing agent to a final dilution of 1 part to 250. The function of the reagent system is to eliminate RBCs and maintain the WBCs in a fixed state.

Basophil

In the basophil method whole blood is diluted to a final dilution of 1 part to 125 in a lysing reagent which eliminates red blood cells, stroma and the cytoplasm of all white blood cells other than basophils through the use of an acid surfactant.

Eosinophil

Whole blood is diluted in a third channel to a final dilution of 1 part in 250 in a reagent in which red blood cells and all white blood cells other than eosinophils are hemolyzed through the use of an alkaline surfactant.

Reticulocytes

The Sysmex R-1000 series systems automate the dilution, staining and counting of reticulocytes and the RBCs. Thus both proportional and absolute reticulocyte counts are produced. For this method a fluorescent dye (auramine-O) is used to stain the RNA. The reticulocytes are then detected on the basis of the fluorescent signal size after being illuminated by an argon laser in a sheath stream flow cell.

TOA measurement technology

The measurement technology consists of a hemoglobin colorimeter at 555 nm and three different types of aperture impedance cell counters.

- A hydrodynamic focused DC aperture impedance counter for RBC/ platelet.
- A multiple detector electrical system (RF/DC) for WBC, and three WBC sub-classes.
- Two non-hydrodynamic focused DC aperture impedance counters for the eosinophil and basophil counts.

The hydrodynamic focused DC cell counter

TOA employs a hydrodynamic focused aperture impedance cell counter for counting and sizing red blood cells and platelets. In this cell counter an aperture dimension of 50 μm in diameter is used. However, the effective sensing volume is further reduced by the sheath reagent. A total equivalent to 0.0234 μl of specimen is analyzed in the RBC/platelet channel yielding approximately 100 000 RBCs and 5000 platelets counted for normal specimens. In the case of a low platelet count the counting period is extended by a factor of two.

The RF/DC cell counter

A second type of aperture impedance system for WBCs in which simultaneous measurements are made both at direct current and at radio frequency on each cell passing through the aperture. The impedance at the RF frequency is reduced relative to the DC impedance for cells with substantial internal structure. Thus, the structure of the granulocytes, and to a lesser extent the monocytes, is distinguishable by comparing the signal amplitude at the two different frequencies. An aperture dimension of 100 μm in diameter is used for this cell counter. Hydrodynamic focusing is not used in the RF/DC cell counter. The RF/DC cell counter is used with the WBC method for distinguishing among white cells, granulocytes, lymphocytes and monocytes. Plate VII shows the cytogram of the RF signal versus the DC signal in the RF/DC aperture impedance cell counter. Also shown are the locations of abnormal cells.

The DC cell counter

Simple DC aperture impedance cell counters without hydrodynamic focusing are used for counting the cells after differential lysis in the basophil and eosinophil channels. A 100 μm aperture is used for counting in these two cell counters.

TOA parameter definition techniques

Discrimination is principally conducted via one dimensional floating (a-posteriori) thresholds called autodiscriminators. In the RBC and platelet method, an autodiscriminator which can range from signal equivalents of 2 to 6 μm^3 is used to discriminate between platelets and noise. A second autodiscriminator which can range from signal equivalents of 12 to 30 μm^3 is used to define the upper limit of platelets, while another autodiscriminator with signal equivalents ranging between 25 μm^3 and 75 μm^3 defines the lower limits of red blood cells. A fourth autodiscriminator ranging from 200 μm^3 to 250 μm^3 defines the upper limit of red blood cells.

The system does not use fitting algorithms for the distributions of either red cells or platelets. The MCV is calculated by the ratio of the sum of weighted RBC signals to the RBC count. The red cell distribution width is calculated nonparametrically from the region in which 68% of the RBC signals fall. The mean platelet volume (MPV) is calculated in a manner analogous to the MCV and the platelet distribution width is calculated nonparametrically by the region defined by the points where the platelet signal histogram falls to 20% of its peak value.

The WBC differential is obtained by combining the results of the three WBC counting channels. The basophil and eosinophil counts are derived from autodiscriminators in their respective channels which separate the unlysed cells from the remainder of the leukocytes. The RF/DC cell counter analyzes the total population of nucleated cells. Figure 3.12 shows the presumed location of the WBC cell populations in a cytogram in which the Y axis is proportional to the RF signal amplitude and the X axis is proportional to the DC signal. The RF/DC counter uses a-posteriori thresholds in two dimensions (angular lines in a cytogram) to discriminate between noise and the major cell populations (lymphocytes, monocytes and granulocytes) as shown in Figure 3.12. Neutrophils are then calculated by subtracting the counts of eosinophils and basophils from the count of total granulocytes derived in the RF/DC counter.

An equivalent of 1 μl of specimen is analyzed in the WBC and eosinophil methods while an equivalent of 2 μl of specimen is analyzed in the basophil method.

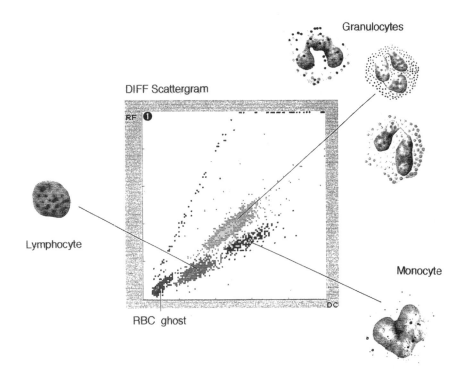

Figure 3.12 Normal patterns on DIFF scattergram (Sysmex Corporation, Long Grove, IL, USA)

THE BAYER (TECHNICON) SYSTEMS

Bayer sampling

The Technicon H*1 system which was introduced in 1985 was the first of the current generation of automated cell counters. The original system required manually mixed open tube specimen containers. Since that time Bayer has introduced enhancements and the Bayer systems now offer both automated sampling and sampling from sealed manually presented specimen containers. In the Bayer automated sampler, specimens in their closed collection tubes are inserted into approximately 100 links of a continuous belt which transports them to the aspiration station. Specimens are mixed by rocking for approximately three minutes before aspiration. The Bayer sampler features the ability to interchange randomly the use of several different specimen containers by providing different adapters which can be attached to the specimen belt.

The manual samplers are available in either closed or open tube versions. In either case, the operator must mix the specimen before presenting it to the aspiration station.

The aspiration station draws about 150 μl of specimen into a shear valve with four isolation chambers. Two of the chambers (RBC/platelet, hemoglobin) isolate 2 μl of specimen while the other two (WBC 1, WBC 2) are 12 μl in volume.

The Bayer systems also feature the ability to analyze a prepared sample by direct aspiration. Recently (1993) Bayer introduced a method by which the percentage of reticulocytes can be determined with the H*3 system by direct aspiration after manual dilution and staining.

Bayer processing methods

In the Bayer automated cell counting systems, the blood specimen is divided into four separate channels:

1. Hemoglobin.
2. RBC and platelets.
3. WBC peroxidase.
4. WBC basophils.

The following paragraphs briefly describe the sample processing methods used for each channel.

Hemoglobin

The hemoglobin method uses a rapid transformation of hemoglobin into a cyanated product which is accomplished in less than 40 seconds as opposed to the three minutes required by the ICSH method. In the Bayer hemoglobin method, 2 μl of whole blood is diluted one part to 250 with a hemoglobin diluent. The diluent contains a surfactant and potassium cyanide which are dissolved in an alkaline borate solution at pH 11.3. The surfactant causes hemolysis of the red blood cells plus emulsification of all cellular debris and plasma lipids. This results in a reaction mixture that is essentially free of turbidity. Following the release of hemoglobin by hemolysis, the combined action of an alkaline pH and surfactant results in rapid denaturation of the protein with solubilization of the hemes by surfactant micelles. The hemes then undergo air oxidation of ferrous iron to the ferric state and combine with cyanide forming micellized ferriheme. The reaction reaches completion very quickly and absorbance is measured at approximately 546 nm 25 seconds after initiation of the reaction on the lower (60 per hour) sampling rate systems and 12 seconds after initiation on the higher sampling rate systems. Bayer has recently released a cyanide free alternative method similar to the TOA method.

RBC and platelets

The red blood cell and platelet method is a one reagent method. When whole blood is mixed with the RBC diluent, the red cells and platelets are isovolumetrically sphered (Kim and Ornstein, 1983) for more accurate and precise determination of the corpuscular volume and hemoglobin distributions from the optical scatter measurement. From an initial whole blood volume of 2 μl the overall dilution of the specimen in the RBC platelet method is 1 part in 625.

WBC peroxidase

The peroxidase method is used to differentiate lymphocytes, monocytes, neutrophils and eosinophils, and consists of a two step cytochemical reaction utilizing three reagents. The blood specimen is first diluted 1 to 21 with peroxidase diluent 1, which contains sodium dodecyl sulfate, formaldehyde and sorbitol in 100 millimolar phosphate buffer at pH 7.2. Formaldehyde and sorbitol combine to yield a hypertonic solution which causes dehydration of the white blood cells. Sodium dodecyl sulfate along with the thermal stress imposed by the temperature gradient causes the lysis of the red blood cells. Formaldehyde fixes the white blood cells and their intracellular enzymes. The hypertonic environment causes some shrinkage and crenation of the white cells which increases the refractive index of the cells and enhances the detection of lymphocytes.

In the second step peroxidase diluents 2 and 3 are added bringing the dye (4-chloro-1-naphthol) and the substrate (hydrogen peroxide) separately to the reaction. The stain is produced by the peroxidase activity which is in the granules of the peroxidase containing white blood cells. The reaction catalyzed by the cellular peroxidase precipitates the dye into a dark precipitate which remains within the cytoplasm of the cell. The amount of staining is determined by the concentration of peroxidase within the cell. Hence, lymphocytes which contain no peroxidase do not precipitate in the stain, monocytes which contain small amounts of peroxidase precipitate some stain, and neutrophils and eosinophils which contain substantial amounts of peroxidase precipitate substantial amounts of stain.

WBC basophils

In the basophil lobularity method whole blood is mixed with a reagent consisting of a combination of acid and surfactant. The red blood cells are hemolyzed and the cytoplasm is stripped from all white cells except basophils. Thus, after reaction three classes of cells may be recognized: intact basophils, polymorphonuclear WBCs, and mononuclear WBCs.

Reticulocytes

For the reticulocyte method the specimen is reacted in a manual preparation step with an absorbing dye (Oxazine-750) to color the RNA. The method also employs a surfactant to isovolumetrically sphere the RBC so that the distributions of cell volume and cell hemoglobin concentration can be obtained together with the reticulocyte count.

Bayer measurement technology

The Bayer measurements are made with a hemoglobin colorimeter at 546 nm, and two separate multiple detector optical cell counters identified principally by the optical source.

1. A white light counter.
2. A laser counter.

The white light lamp counter

The white light counter measures the intensity of light scattered and of light absorbed by each cell after staining with the peroxidase method. Illumination is via a tungsten lamp whose light is focused to a rectangular slit of 25 μm height. Hydrodynamic focusing is used with a sample stream of 40 μm in diameter and a sample flow rate of 0.1 μm per minute. These dimensions define the sensing volume as a cylinder of 40 μm in diameter and 25 μm in length. The collected light is then split by a dichroic mirror (reflects one color while transmitting another) with equal reflectance and transmittance at 700 μm. The longer wavelengths are directed to the scatter detector while the shorter wavelengths are directed to the absorption detector.

The cell counter is used to count and classify cells after being stained in the peroxidase method. The resulting signal distribution for a normal specimen is shown in Figure 3.13 as a cytogram in which the light scatter signal is shown as the Y axis and the light absorption signal as the X axis. It can be seen that distinct clusters are formed for each of the four cell types classified by this counter (lymphocytes, neutrophils, eosinophils and monocytes).

The laser cell counter

In the laser cell counter, excitation is with a helium neon laser at 632.8 nm. Measurements are made of the intensity of light scattered by

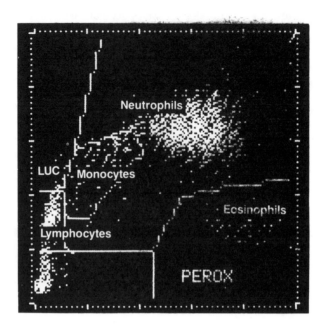

Figure 3.13 Cytogram for the Bayer peroxidase channel. Light scatter signal
is Y axis, while the light absorption signal is the X axis

each cell into two angular regions, 2 degrees to 3 degrees and 5 degrees
to 10 degrees. Hydrodynamic focusing is used with the sample stream
of 20 μm diameter and a processing rate of 0.1 μl per minute. The illumination optics focuses the laser light into a rectangular slit whose
height is 15 μm. Thus the sensing volume consists of a cylinder of
20 μm in diameter and 15 μm in length. The Bayer Laser Cell counter
is used twice for each blood specimen. First as the cell counter for the
Bayer RBC and platelet method, and second for the Bayer basophil
method. Figures 3.14a and 3.14b show the cytograms obtained on the
Bayer systems for the RBC platelet method and the basophil method
respectively where the Y axis is the low angle scatter and the X axis is
the high angle scatter. Figure 3.15 shows the transformation map
(based on the Mie theory) which is used to convert the RBC cytogram
into cell volume and cell hemoglobin concentration.

Bayer parameter definition techniques

Bayer uses a-priori discrimination for the CBC parameters and a-posteriori discrimination for the leukocyte differential. In the Bayer

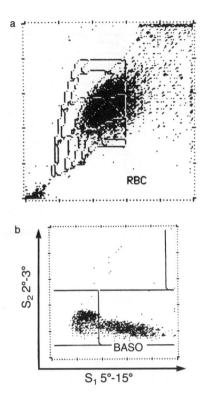

Figure 3.14 Bayer laser cell counter: (a) normal red blood cell cytogram (b) cytogram obtained when basophil effluent is analyzed. (Bayer Diagnostics, Tarrytown, NY, USA)

systems red cells and platelets are discriminated on the basis of low angle scatter signal along with a fixed threshold placed at a signal equivalent of approximately 30 μm. Platelets are discriminated from noise on the basis of a fixed threshold of a signal equivalent of 2 μm. The accumulated platelet counts are then fitted to a log normal curve and the fitted curve used to calculate the mean platelet volume and the platelet distribution width.

The two angular scatter signals are combined to analyze the size of the red blood cells. To perform this analysis a transformation of the two signals is made via a specific algorithm based on the Mie theory into a space in which cell size and cell hemoglobin concentration are orthogonal axes. The resulting distributions are then fitted to normal distributions along each of these axes. The red cell distribution width (RDW)

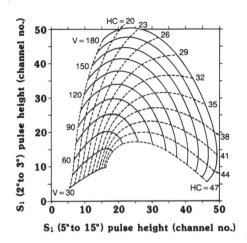

Figure 3.15 Transformation map used in Bayer System to transform scattered light intensity to cell volume and cell hemoglobin (Bayer Diagnostics, Tarrytown, NY, USA)

and the hemoglobin distribution width (HDW) are obtained from the standard deviations of the fitted curves.

In the peroxidase method a two dimensional Gaussian cluster analysis algorithm is used to define the clusters for each cell type which is classified and to set curvilinear a-posteriori thresholds to isolate the clusters. Fixed a-priori thresholds are used to discriminate noise. Cells are classified into five categories (neutrophils, lymphocytes, monocytes, eosinophils and large unstained (LUC) cells). The LUC cells are thus defined as cells which are larger than normal lymphocytes but have no peroxidase activity. Since this definition excludes all normal cells the LUC count is used as a flag for variant lymphocytes and other abnormal cells.

In the basophil channels a-priori thresholds are used to discriminate noise from leukocytes and "stripped leukocytes" from basophils. A one dimensional a-posteriori threshold is used to analyze the leukocytes from which the cytoplasm has been stripped and separate them into polymorphonuclear cells and mononuclear cells. Flagging for immature granulocytes is derived by comparing the counts of peroxidase positive neutrophils and eosinophils to the counts of polynuclear cells in the basophil lobularity channel. A specific flag for blast cells is also derived from the basophil channel. Figures 3.16a and 3.16b show examples of the discrimination algorithms and the locations of the cell populations on the peroxidase and basophil cytograms.

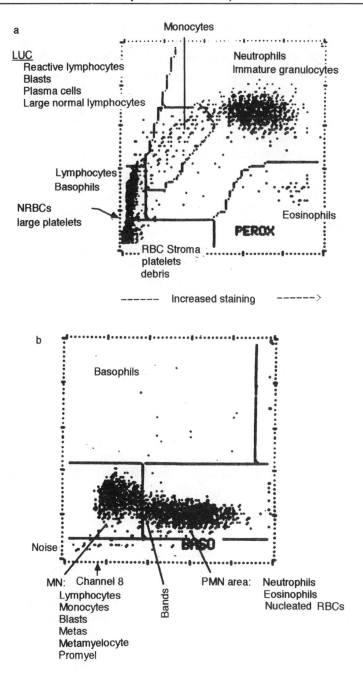

Figure 3.16 Example of the Bayer cell classification scheme: a) peroxidase cytogram, b) basophil cytogram. (Bayer Diagnostics, Tarrytown, NY, USA)

The Bayer systems report a six parameter differential including the five mature cell types plus the LUC count from the peroxidase channel.

Qualitatively abnormal specimen flagging is based on the analysis of the distributions of the following cell types:

1. Platelet size distribution.
2. Peroxidase positive cells distributed in absorption.
3. Peroxidase negative cell distribution in scatter.
4. Mononuclear cells in the basophil channel.

THE ABBOTT SYSTEMS

Abbott sampling

The Abbott systems aspirate from an automatically mixed and presented specimen container (Cell-Dyn 3500 and Cell-Dyn 3000) or from a manually mixed and presented specimen (Cell-Dyn 1600 and Cell-Dyn 1700). The systems can accommodate either closed or open specimen containers. In either case, the specimen is aspirated into a shear valve which isolates three sample segments. A 20 μl sample is isolated for the determination of hemoglobin (and WBC count), a 0.6 μl sample is isolated for the sizing and counting of RBCs and platelets, and a 32 μl segment is isolated for the WBC differential.

Abbott methods

The automated cell counters utilize up to three automated methods: one for determination of hemoglobin, one for sizing and counting of cells (platelets, RBCs and WBCs) and a third for the differential leukocyte count.

Hemoglobin

The hemoglobin reagent is specifically formulated to hemolyze red blood cells and complete the conversion to hemoglobin cyanide. The Abbot hemoglobin method works by diluting the 20 μl segment isolated by the shear valve in a single step to a final dilution of 1 part of blood to 300 with the hemoglobin reagent. Abbott has also recently released an alternative cyanide free hemoglobin method.

RBC and platelets

In the RBC and platelet counting method, whole blood is diluted in a single step to a final dilution of 1 part in 12 500 in an isotonic diluent;

100 μl of this dilution is measured. Thus approximately 40 thousand RBCs are analyzed for a normal specimen. In the case of low platelet count the counting interval is extended by a factor two.

WBC

A total dilution of 1 part in 51 is made in a single step with a proprietary reagent whose function is to maintain the white cells as close to their native state as possible while eliminating the signals from red blood cells. Approximately 1 μl of equivalent specimen is analyzed. Thus, the number of cells classified for the WBC differential is roughly equal to the white blood cell count in cells per μl. However, if the count is less than 4000 the counting interval is extended by a factor of two.

Abbott measurement technology

The measurement technology consists of a hemoglobin colorimeter at 540 nm, two DC aperture impedance cell counters (one for the WBC count and one for the RBC and platelet channel) and a multiple detector optical cell counter.

The aperture impedance cell counter

In the aperture impedance cell counter an aperture of 100 μm in diameter and 70 μm in length is used for the WBC count, while an aperture of 60 μm in diameter is used for counting and sizing RBC and platelets. The aperture impedance detector does not use backsweeping or hydrodynamic focusing, but a patented transducer device called the Von Behrens plate transducer is used to prevent cells from re-entering the sensing zone. Pulse width editing is used to eliminate signals from cells with nonaxial trajectories.

The Abbott optical cell counter

The Abbott optical cell counter is used for the white blood cell methodology. In the optical cell counter, hydrodynamic focusing is used to reduce the sample stream to 25 μm in diameter. A laser is used as the optical light source and each cell is individually characterized by four specific angles of light scatter. The light source is a polarized five milliwatt helium neon laser at 6328 nm. The laser head is oriented so that the plane of polarization is vertical. As the light passes from the laser to the flow cell, the laser beam is shaped and focused to an elliptical pattern whose minor axis is perpendicular to the direction of the cells flowing by. A white blood cell entering the focused laser beam will scatter light in all directions because the wavelength of light is small compared to the blood cell size. Specific portions of the scattered light are collected for use in the WBC differential.

Two silicon photodiode detectors measure the light scattered at low angles with respect to the laser beam. One of these detectors detects the light scattered from 1 degree to 3 degrees (called 0° scatter) which is mainly affected by the size of the cell, and the other detects the light scattered from 3 degrees to 11 degrees (called 10° scatter) which is mainly a function of the internal structure of the cell. Two photomultiplier detectors measure the light scattered at 90 degrees to the laser beam. One detector has a polarizer oriented in the direction of the polarization of the laser light. The other detector has a polarizer oriented at 90 degrees to the direction of original laser light polarization and is sensitive to the scattered light which has been depolarized by the interaction with the blood cells. The optical cell counter generates the primary white blood cell count and differential using the proprietary Multi-Angle-Polarized-Scatter Separation (MAPSS) methodology. The two low angle photodiodes form the primary basis for discrimination. Figure 3.17a shows a cytogram of the light scattered from 1 to 3 degrees versus the light scattered from 3 to 11 degrees on a normal specimen indicating the locations of the normal cell populations. Individual clusters of lymphocytes, monocytes and neutrophils are apparent. The two detectors at 90 degrees are used for discriminating among the other white cells. Figure 3.17b shows the cytogram of the polarized versus the depolarized scattered light at 90 degrees, indicating the locations of eosinophils and basophils. Plate VIII shows the output distribution of white blood cells from a normal specimen analyzed on the Cell-Dyn 3500 system.

Abbott parameter definition techniques

In the Abbott system, discrimination in the RBC/platelet channel is made via one dimensional floating (a-posteriori) thresholds placed in the valleys between the platelets and the noise or the RBC. The platelet and RBC histograms are both fitted to a log normal distribution to obtain size parameters including: MCV, RDW, mean platelet volume, platelet distribution width, and platelet crit. Additional qualitative flags are obtained by monitoring the valleys between platelets and noise or RBC.

Abbott employs the MAPSS method of discrimination to obtain the white blood cell differential parameters from the signals of the optical cell counter. Five sub-types of white blood cells are obtained in the Abbott systems by combining the results of four a-posteriori one dimensional thresholding on each of the four optical scatter measurements. In

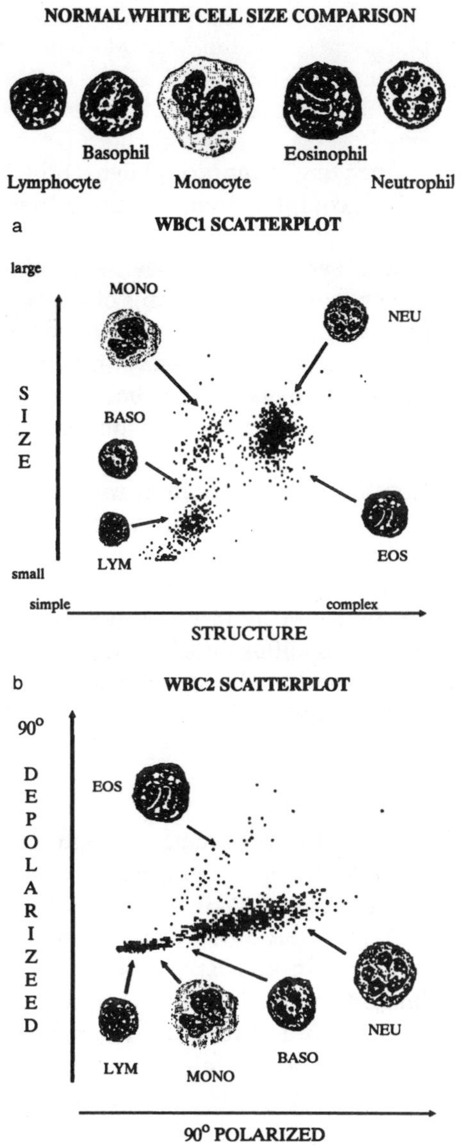

NORMAL WHITE CELL SIZE COMPARISON

Lymphocyte   Basophil   Monocyte   Eosinophil   Neutrophil

a   **WBC1 SCATTERPLOT**

large

S
I
Z
E

MONO

NEU

BASO

LYM

EOS

small

simple   complex

STRUCTURE

b   **WBC2 SCATTERPLOT**

90°

D
E
P
O
L
A
R
I
Z
E
E
D

EOS

LYM   MONO   BASO   NEU

90° POLARIZED

Figure 3.17   Example of the Abbott cell classification scheme: a) low angle vs high angle, b) polarized vs de-polarized. (Abbott Diagnostics, Abbott Park, IL, USA)

addition, qualitative flags are automatically generated to alert the operator when any of the four histograms' analysis does not meet preset conditions.

THE ROCHE SYSTEMS

Roche sampling

As indicated in the product line summary above, the Roche systems are available in alternative configurations with either automated or manual sampling.

In the Roche automated sampler, 32 closed specimen containers are disposed radially on a vertical wheel. Mixing of the specimens prior to aspiration is accomplished by rotating the sampler wheel.

Manual sampling offers the option of sampling from either closed or open specimen containers after they have been manually mixed. The Roche systems also offer the opportunity to sample pre-diluted and pre-mixed capillary specimens.

In the automated sampler the specimen is aspirated into a multiport shear valve in which up to three samples are isolated. One 25 μl sample is isolated for the determination of both hemoglobin and the RBC/platelet channel, a 25 μl sample for the main WBC differential and a 15 μl sample for the counting of basophils. In the Roche systems which perform only a limited differential a single 25 μl sample is isolated and the WBC count is obtained from the same sample following the determination of hemoglobin.

Roche methods

The systems use up to a total of four methods: one for hemoglobin, one for counting red blood cells and platelets, one for counting leukocytes and differentiating four classes of WBC, and one for the independent counting of basophils. A pre-dilution in isotonic saline of 1/200 is performed for both the hemoglobin and RBC/platelet methods. A separate WBC count is available from the hemoglobin channel and for the systems with a partial or limited differential the cell size data from this channel is used.

Hemoglobin

In the hemoglobin channel the pre-diluted specimen is brought to a final dilution of 1:240 with a lysing reagent which also contains cyanide. RBCs are lysed and the hemoglobin is converted to a stable cyanated form.

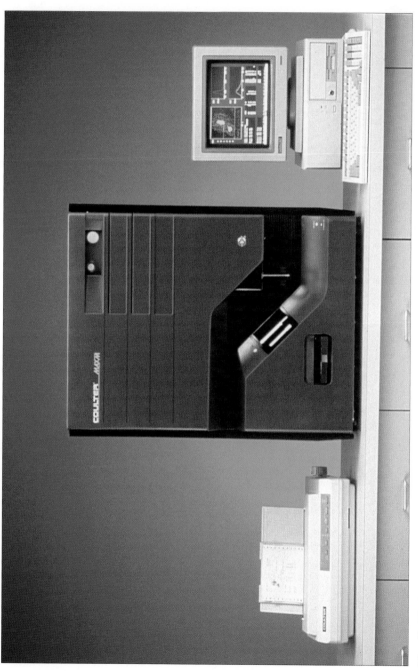

Plate I The MAXM system. Courtesy of the Coulter Corp., Hialeah, FL, USA

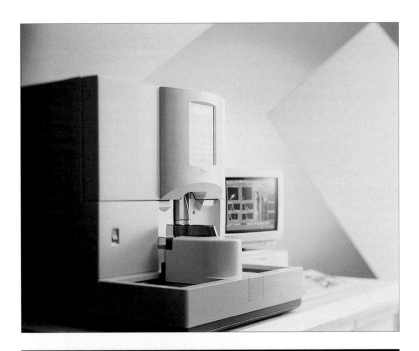

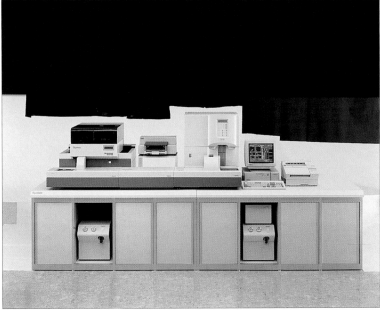

Plate II The SE-9000 instrument: (above) as a stand-alone instrument; (below) integrated into the SE-Alpha Hematology system. Courtesy of Sysmex Corp., Long Grove, IL, USA

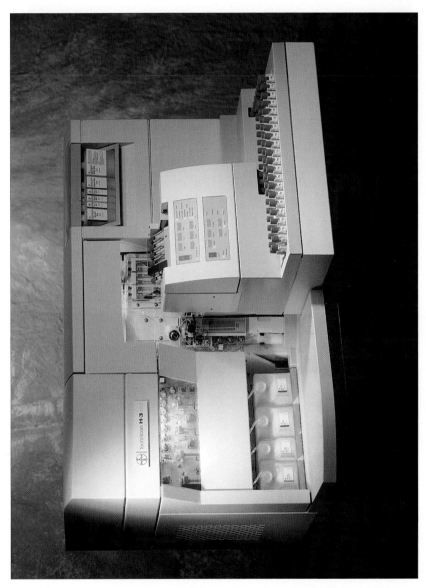

Plate III The Technicon H*3 system. Courtesy of Bayer Diagnostics, Tarreytown, NY, USA

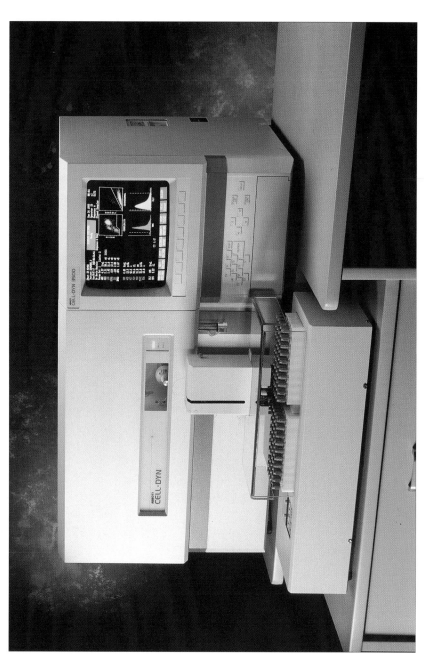

Plate IV The CD-3500 System. Courtesy of Abbott Diagnostics Division, Santa Clara, CA, USA

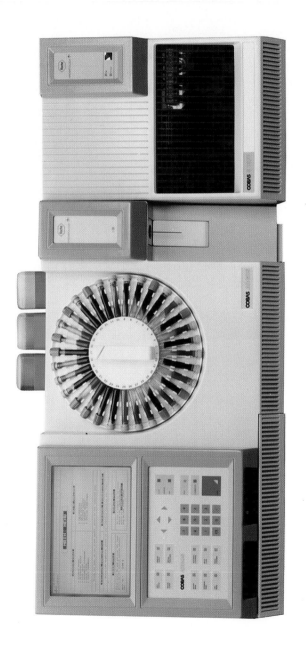

Plate V The fully automated Argos System. Courtesy of Roche Diagnostics, Branchburg, NJ, USA

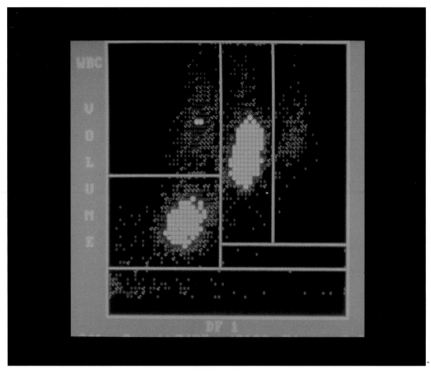

Plate VI Example of the output from the MAXM system showing the distribution of leukocytes. Courtesy of the Coulter Corp., Hialeah, FL, USA

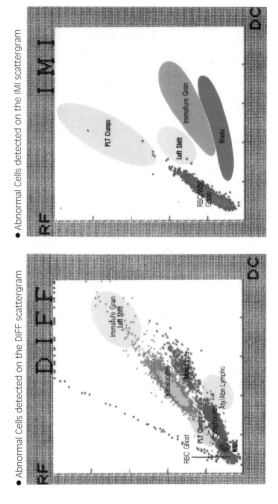

● Abnormal Cells detected on the DIFF scattergram

● Abnormal Cells detected on the IMI scattergram

Plate VII An example of the normal and abnormal white blood cell classification with the SE-9000 system. Courtesy of Sysmex Corp., Long Grove, IL, USA

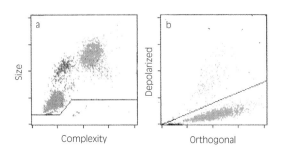

Plate VIII An example of the white blood cell classification on the CD-3500 system. Courtesy of Abbott Diagnostics Division, Santa Clara, CA, USA

RBC/platelet

In the RBC/platelet channel a second dilution with isotonic saline deals a total dilution of 1 part in 10 000.

WBC

In the main WBC differential channel blood specimens are also diluted in two steps and mixed with a proprietary reagent to a final dilution of 1:240. The function of the reagent is to destroy the red blood cells and fix the white blood cells with minimum distortion. Eosinophil granules are stained with this reagent to enhance their separation from neutrophils in the cell counter.

WBC basophil

Basophils are diluted in a single step to 1:133 in another proprietary reagent that destroys red blood cells and lyses all of the white blood cells except for the basophils.

Roche measurement technology

The measurement technology consists of a hemoglobin colorimeter at 540 nm, two aperture impedance cell counters and a multiple detector combination of aperture impedance and optical absorption.

The aperture impedance cell counters

Three DC aperture impedance cell counters are used in the Roche systems with separate apertures: a 100 μm aperture without hydrodynamic focusing is used for counting white cells, a 50 μm aperture without hydrodynamic focusing is used for counting and sizing red cells and platelets, and an 80 μm aperture without hydrodynamic focusing is used for counting basophils.

Combined transducer optical counter

In the combined transducer optical counter an aperture impedance detector of 60 μm in diameter is coupled with optical absorption. Hydrodynamic focusing is used in this counter. Figure 3.18 illustrates the Roche combined transducer cell counter. The patented flow cell uses a double sheathing principle to ensure a narrow and even stream as the cells pass through the sizing aperture (C) and then the optical measurement zone. The hydrodynamic focusing limits the sensing volume, thus

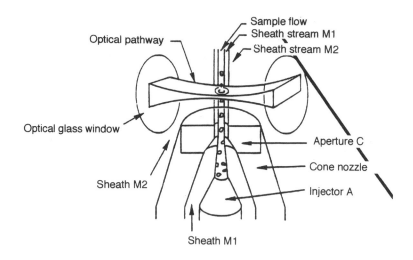

Figure 3.18   The Roche combined transducer flow cell. Cells focused hydraulically by sheath M1 are sized in the DC aperture C then refocused by sheath M2 into the optical pathway (Roche Diagnostics, Brancheburg, NJ, USA)

mitigating the increased volume created by the sequential detectors, and ensuring that the cells flow through one by one for accurate counting, sizing and optical measurement.

The first measurement (aperture impedance) is taken for count and size as the cells pass through the 60 μm aperture. The second measurement taken is the optical transmission to obtain information on the internal structure of the cells. The results of these measurements for a normal specimen are used to develop a cytogram as illustrated in Plate IV where the aperture impedance measurement is shown as the X axis, and the optical absorption measurement as the Y axis.

Roche parameter definition techniques

The red blood cells and platelets are discriminated with a one dimensional floating (a-posteriori) threshold on the signals obtained from the DC aperture impedance cell counter. A fixed threshold at a nominal value of 2 μm^3 cubed is used to discriminate between platelets and noise. Since hydrodynamic focusing is not used in this channel, elimination of nonaxial trajectories and recirculation is done with pulse editing techniques.

The red cell distribution width is determined from the standard deviation of the RBC signal amplitudes and reported as a percentage of the mean cell volume. The mean platelet volume and platelet size distribution are determined by analysis of the platelet signal amplitudes

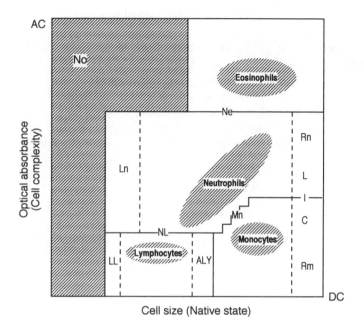

Figure 3.19 Morphological flag regions (COBAS HELIOS/COBAS ARGOS – Roche Diagnostics, Brancheburg, NJ). ALY, atypical lymphocytes; LIC, large immature cells. Morphological flags: LL, left lymphocyte; NL, neutrophil/lymphocyte; Ln, left neutrophil; Mn, monocyte/neutrophil; Rn, right neutrophil; Rm, right monocyte; Ne, neutrophil/eosinophil; No, noise

without fitting. The distribution width is simply taken as the signal amplitude range including 70% of the platelet signals.

Six individual WBC classes are created by two one dimensional fixed (a-priori) thresholds applied to the cytogram formed in the main WBC differential channel (Figure 3.19). The six classes consist of four mature WBC sub-classes (neutrophils, monocytes, lymphocytes and eosinophils) plus two additional classes. The two additional classes of abnormal cells define atypical lymphoid cells and large immature cells. Basophils are counted separately by a floating (a-posteriori) one dimensional threshold operating in the separate basophil channel. The Roche differential reports seven sub-types of WBC including the counts of the atypical lymphoid cells and large immature cells. However, counts of the two abnormal sub-classes are also included in the count of the five major classes of leukocytes. Additional qualitative flags for abnormal specimens are also obtained from the analysis of the WBC differential cytogram in the regions denoted as LN, LL, and interference with the thresholds Ne and Mn (Figure 3.19).

COMPARISON OF METHODS

We have seen in the previous sections how each of several multipara-meter cell counters functions to obtain a CBC, including a full five part differential, plus additional qualitative flags, and cell size parameters. It was apparent in these descriptions that although most of the reported results (parameters) are the same, the method by which they are obtained on one system may be quite different than on another. Therefore, it is useful to summarize the information by comparing the methods used by the different manufacturers for obtaining each of the reported parameters.

SPECIMEN DIVISION AND DILUTION

Each of the cell counting systems which perform a complete WBC differ-ential divides the specimen into a minimum of three parallel sample preparation channels. Table 3.2 summarizes the sample division and preparation for each of the systems discussed and compares them. It is seen that there is variation in the number of channels and the number of reagents required for sample processing. As indicated in Chapter 2 the systems which use the least reagents and channels for the WBC differential (Coulter and Abbott) utilize more complex detectors, while the systems with the most complex sample preparation (TOA) employ the least complex detectors. Finally, since some of the systems use hydrodynamic focusing, additional reagents are required for the liquid sheath.

Table 3.2 Comparison of full differential systems

Manufacturer	System	Samples per hour	Analysis channels	Active reagents	Other reagents
Coulter	MAXM	75	3	4	1
Coulter	STKS	109	3	4	1
TOA	NE-8000	120	5	6	3
TOA	NE-9000	120	7	6	3
Bayer	H*1, H*3 RTC	60	4	6	4
Bayer	H*2, H*3 RTX	102	4	6	4
Abbott	CD3500	100	3	4	1
Roche	ARGOS	120	4	4	3
Roche	HELIOS	70	4	4	3

*Sheath and cleaning.

Table 3.3. Comparison of methods for hemoglobin

Item	Coulter	TOA	Bayer	Abbott	Roche
Sample dilution	1:251	1:500	1:250	1:300	1:240
Identification method	Cyanmet-Hb	SLS-met-Hb	Cyanmet-Hb*	Cyanmet-Hb*	Cyanmet-Hb
Detection method	Absorb at 525 nm	Absorb at 540 nm	Absorb at 546 nm	Absorb at 540 nm	Absorb at 540 nm
Combine with WBC	Yes	No	No	Yes	Yes

*Non-cyanide method optional.
SLS-met Hb, sodium laurel sulfate complex with hemoglobin.

HEMOGLOBIN

The methods for obtaining the total blood hemoglobin concentration are the most similar of all. Table 3.3 summarizes the comparison between manufacturers for the method of obtaining total hemoglobin. Each of the analyzers dilutes the specimen by approximately 1:250 in a reagent which is designed to destroy the red cell membrane and convert the hemoglobin to a single stable form. Results are then read with an absorption filter photometer (colorimeter) at approximately 540 nm. The only exception is TOA which employs a total dilution of 1:500. Each of the manufacturers with the exception of TOA also attempts to convert the hemoglobin to a cyanated form before measurement in agreement with the ICSH reference method. However, concern with the hazards posed by cyanide in the waste stream of the cell counter has prompted the development of non-cyanide methods by TOA, Abbott and Bayer.

Recent TOA systems employ the non-cyanide (SLS) method exclusively, while the non-cyanide method is offered optionally by Bayer and Abbott.

RBC/PLATELET

Table 3.4 summarizes the comparisons of some of the important parameters regarding the measurement of RBC counts, platelet counts and the associated size parameters.

Counting

The methodology employed by the manufacturers for obtaining the RBC and platelet counts and size parameters is similar in that the data is universally obtained in a single channel which accomplishes the count-

Table 3.4 Comparison of methods for counting RBCs/platelet (PLT)

Item	Coulter	TOA	Bayer	Abbott	Roche
Sample dilution	1:6251	1:500	1:625	1:12500	1:10000
Identification method	Preserve	Preserve	Sphere	Preserve	Preserve
Detection method	DC imped.	DC imped.	Optical	DC imped.	DC imped.
Discriminator PLT/noise	Curve fitting	Floating 1 dim.	Fixed 1 dim.	Floating 1 dim.	Fixed 1 dim.
Discriminator RBC/platelet	Floating 1 dim.	Floating 1 dim.	Floating 2 dim.	Floating 1 dim.	Floating 1 dim.
No. of cells counted (normal)	50 K RBC 3 K PLT	110 K RBC 6 K PLT	45 K RBC 2.5 K PLT	40 K RBC 2 K PLT	?
Extended count	Yes	Yes	No	Yes	No
Red cell size*	RDW (SD)	RDW (SD) RDW (CV)	RDW (CV) HDW	RDW (CV)	RDW (CV)
Platelet size*	MPV (log)	MPV PDW P-LCR	MPV PDW P-crit	MPB (log) PDW (log) P-crit	MPV PDW
Hydraulic control	Backswept aperture	Hydro-dynamic focus	Hydro-dynamic focus	Von Behrens plate	Pulse edit

HDW, the distribution of Hb content.
P-LCR, the platelet large cell ratio.
*Unless noted, parameters based on normal model.

ing and sizing of RBCs and platelets at the same time and same dilution. Bayer uses optical scatter whereas all the others use aperture impedance. All manufacturers discriminate between the two cell types simply on basis of signal amplitude in this channel. However, a glance at Table 3.4 will show that a wide range of dilution is employed. This is necessary to reduce coincidence in the various cell counters which have different sensing volumes. TOA and Bayer use hydrodynamic focusing to obtain a small detection volume and consequently use a much lower dilution. The other three manufacturers use aperture impedance sensors without hydrodynamic focusing of approximately 50 μm diameter and 50 μm length. These manufactures must also confront the problems of nonaxial flow and potential recirculation errors. Coulter uses pulse width editing to eliminate the effect of the nonaxial cells from the sizing calculation and a backswept aperture to eliminate recirculation. Abbott uses pulse editing for nonaxial trajectories and the proprietary

Von Behrens plate to eliminate recirculation. Roche employs a complex pulse editing system for elimination of both the errors due to recirculation and nonaxial trajectories.

One problem which results from counting both platelets and RBCs in the same dilution is the required dynamic range of counting (from low platelet counts to high RBC counts) which approaches 100 to 1. This causes all of the manufacturers to insert a coincidence correction for the RBC count, with the attendant problems of two class coincidence correction. In addition, three of the manufacturers (Coulter, TOA and Abbott) extend the counting period when the platelet count is low.

Another problem which is confronted in the combined RBC/platelet channel is the discrimination between platelets and spurious noise pulses. Bayer and Roche use fixed (a-priori) thresholds placed at a nominal value of 2 μm^3. The other three manufacturers use a-posteriori discrimination techniques. TOA and Abbott use floating thresholds. Coulter uses a curve fitting algorithm and integrates the fitted curve to obtain the platelet count.

Sizing

With the exception of Bayer each of the manufacturers obtains a size dependent signal with aperture impedance detection after preparing the cells by simply diluting the anticoagulated blood in an isotonic diluent at a pH of approximately 7.4. Bayer spheres the red blood cells at constant volume and measures the size with a two angle optical scatter system. Conversion, from the signal size in the two optical sensing detectors, into red blood cell size is made by using a special algorithm based on the optical scattering of spherical dielectric particles.

The red cell distribution width is universally obtained as the standard deviation (central 68%) of the red cell size signals. However, it is alternatively reported as percentage variation (CV) or as the standard deviation (SD) in femtoliters. In some systems both numbers are reported.

Platelet size is obtained in all systems directly from the detector signal amplitude. Four of the manufacturers use aperture impedance detectors while Bayer uses a single optical scatter determination. It is widely believed that one action of the anticoagulant EDTA is to transform the platelet shape to roughly spherical. Thus, a major sizing problem (shape) is eliminated. However, platelets (unlike RBCs) contain internal elements which have different effects on the optical and aperture impedance detection systems. Further, the platelet is generally subject to in-vitro storage effects which modify both its size and shape. These effects are also detected differently with the different sensor systems (Jackson and Carter, 1993).

Platelet mean size is variably reported in terms of normal or log normal size parameters. Coulter calculates the mean platelet volume and platelet distribution width as the results (mean and geometric standard deviation) of the log normal fitting algorithm used to obtain the platelet count. Bayer and Abbott also use log normal fitting programs to obtain the platelet size distribution, but report the platelet mean volume and standard deviation in terms of the equivalent normal distribution. TOA and Roche do not fit the platelet signal distribution but obtain the platelet distribution width directly from boundaries placed on the signal amplitude histogram. TOA takes as a boundary the point at which the platelet histogram has fallen to 20% of its peak height, while Roche takes the boundaries that include the central 70% of the histogram signals.

NEUTROPHILS

Table 3.5 compares some of the important parameters in the determination of the neutrophil count. Discrimination of the neutrophils on the basis of their granularity is uniform. Two of the manufacturers (Bayer and Roche) recognize the neutrophil granules in absorbed light. In the Bayer system the cells are stained while in the Roche system they are not. Abbott and Coulter also note the effect of the granular structure optically but measure the effect on the scattered light. Two manufac-

Table 3.5 Comparison of methods for counting neutrophils

Item	Coulter	TOA	Bayer	Abbott	Roche
Sample dilution	1:50	1:250	1:52	1:51	1:240
Identification method	Preserve granular	Preserve granular	Stain granules	Preserve granular	Preserve granular
Detection method	VCS	RF imped. vs DC imped	Scatter vs absorb.	MAPSS	Imped. vs absorb.
Discriminator	Floating 3 × 1 dim.	Floating 2 × 1 dim.	Cluster analysis	Floating 2 × 2 dim.	Fixed 2 × 1 dim.
No. of cells counted	WBC/μl	WBC/μl	WBC/μl	WBC/μl	WBC/μl
Other				Extend if WBC < 4000	

MAPSS, multi-angle-polarized-scatter separation contained in two 2 dim. analyses: 90° scatter vs 0° scatter and 90° scatter polarized vs 90° scatter depolarized.
VCS, three parameter volume (DC) conductivity (RF) and scatter.

turers (TOA and Coulter) also recognize the presence of granules by direct impact on the electrical detection methodology by noting the changes in the high frequency aperture impedance signal caused by the increased granular structure. Unfortunately, there is less uniformity in the presentation of the cytograms than in the measurements. Bayer, Abbott and Coulter display the size signal amplitude as the Y axis in their cytograms and the granular structure as the X axis. TOA and Roche display the size signal amplitude as the X axis and the structure as the Y axis.

LYMPHOCYTES

Table 3.6 compares the methods used in counting lymphocytes. Recognition of lymphocytes is principally and uniformly obtained from discrimination by means of a single size dependent signal. Thus, lymphocytes are universally defined as small non-granular cells and not as the result of any specific tag. Detection methods vary with three of the manufacturers using principally DC aperture impedance and two of the manufacturers (Bayer and Abbott) using principally low angle scatter.

Although each of the manufacturers flags variant lymphocytes, two of the manufacturers (Roche and Bayer) attempt to sub-classify lympho-

Table 3.6 Comparison of methods for counting lymphocytes

Item	Coulter	TOA	Bayer	Abbott	Roche
Sample dilution	1 : 50	1 : 250	1 : 52	1 : 51	1 : 240
Identification method	Preserve state	Preserve state	Preserve state	Preserve state	Preserve state
Detection method	VCS	RF imped. vs DC imped	Forward vs scatter	MAPSS	DC imped.
Discriminator	Floating 3 × 1 dim.	Floating 2 × 1 dim.	Cluster analysis	Floating 2 × 2 dim.	Fixed 2 × 1 dim.
No. of cells counted	WBC/μl	WBC/μl	WBC/μl	WBC/μl	WBC/μl
Other			LUC	Extend for low WBC	ALY

LUC, large unstained (peroxidase) cells.
ALY, abnormal lymphoid cells.
MAPSS, multi-angle-polarized-scatter separation contained in two 2 dim. analyses: 90° scatter vs 10° scatter and 0° scatter vs 10° scatter.
VCS, three parameter volume (DC) conductivity (RF) and scatter.

cytes by a discriminator sensitive to oversize cells which are not granular. However, they differ in the matter of reporting this information. Bayer adds a sixth differential category, large unstained cells (LUC), while Roche classifies abnormal lymphoid cells (ALY), which are included in the total count of lymphocytes.

MONOCYTES

Table 3.7 compares some important techniques used in counting monocytes by the different manufacturers. Monocytes are discriminated from lymphocytes on the basis of size and from neutrophils on the absence of structure (granules) by all five manufacturers. This apparent uniformity is misleading, however, since as was stated above there is a variation among manufacturers in the methods of measuring both size and structure. Bayer stains the monocytes for peroxidase; the others do not. Thus, the classification of monocytes, which are typically a smaller population lying between neutrophils and lymphocytes, is much less uniform than would appear. This is further complicated by the sub-classification of lymphocytes in the Bayer and Roche systems. Thus the cells included in the abnormal cell classifications (LUC and ALY) may be included variably in the monocyte or leukocyte classifications of the other manufacturers.

Table 3.7 Comparison of methods for counting monocytes

Item	Coulter	TOA	Bayer	Abbott	Roche
Sample dilution	1 : 50	1 : 250	1 : 52	1 : 51	1 : 240
Identification method	Preserve state	Preserve state	Perox. stain granules	Preserve state	Preserve state
Detection method	VCS	RF imped. vs DC imped.	Scatter vs absorb	MAPSS vs scatter	Imped.
Discriminator	Floating 3 × 1 dim.	Floating 2 × 1 dim.	Cluster analysis	Floating 2 × 2 dim.	Fixed 2 × 1 dim.
No. of cells counted	WBC/μl	WBC/μl	WBC/μl	WBC/μl	WBC/μl
Other				Extend if WBC low	

MAPSS is multi-angle-polarized-scatter separation contained in two 2 dim. analyses 90° vs 10° and 10° vs 0°.
VCS, three parameter volume (DC) conductivity (RF) and scatter.

Table 3.8 Comparison of methods for counting eosinophils

Item	Coulter	TOA	Bayer	Abbott	Roche
Sample dilution	1:50	1:250	1:52	1:51	1:240
Identification method	Preserve granular	Selective lysis	Stain granules	Preserve granular	Stain granules
Detection method	VCS	DC imped.	Scatter vs absorb.	MAPSS	Imped. vs absorb.
Discriminator	Floating 2 × 1 dim.	Floating 2 × 1 dim.	Cluster analysis	Floating 2 × 2 dim.	Fixed 2 × 1 dim.
No. of cells counted	WBC/μl	WBC/μl	WBC/μl	WBC/μl	WBC/μl
Other				Extend if WBC < 4000	

MAPSS, multi-angle-polarized-scatter separation contained in two 2 dim. analyses: 90° scatter vs 10° scatter and 90° scatter polarized vs 90° scatter depolarized.
VCS, three parameter volume (DC) conductivity (RF) and scatter.

EOSINOPHILS

Table 3.8 compares the methods used by the different manufacturers for recognizing and counting eosinophils. In most systems eosinophils are also defined by their granules and are discriminated from neutrophils on the signal characteristics from their granules. Abbott uses the depolarization of light by eosinophil granules. In a manner similar to neutrophils two of the manufacturers (Bayer and Roche) recognize the eosinophils by light absorbed after staining the granules while the others do not. However, except for the Roche method the granules are not specifically stained. Thus discrimination between neutrophils and eosinophils is principally made on the physical characteristics (different structure) of their granules. Discrimination of eosinophils from neutrophils would appear to present a difficult challenge due to the smaller relative number of cells typically encountered. However, unlike monocytes the larger granules and heavy granulation is effective in creating a clear separation no matter which detection method is used.

The TOA systems employ an independent channel for counting eosinophils in which the eosinophils are isolated by differential lysis.

Table 3.9   Comparison of methods for counting basophils

Item	Coulter	TOA	Bayer	Abbott	Roche
Sample dilution	1:50	1:125	1:42	1:51	1:133
Identification method	Preserve state	Selective lysis	Selective lysis	Preserve state	Selective lysis
Detection method	VCS	DC imped.	Scatter	MAPSS	DC imped.
Discriminator	Floating 1 dim.	Floating 1 dim.	Fixed 1 dim.	Floating 2 × 2 dim.	Fixed 1 dim.
No. of cells counted	WBC/μl	2 × WBC/μl	WBC/μl	WBC/μl	WBC/μl
Other				Extend if WBC low	

MAPSS, multi-angle-polarized-scatter separation contained in two 2 dim. analyses: 90° scatter vs 10° scatter and 90° scatter polarized vs 90° scatter depolarized.
VCS, three parameter volume (DC), conductivity (RF), and scatter.

BASOPHILS

Table 3.9 compares the methods used by the different manufacturers in identifying and counting basophils. The difference in methodology is most apparent for the basophil. Three of the five manufacturers use selective lysis to isolate basophils while the other two use the difference in the physical characteristics (structure) of their granules. This is made further diverse by noting that of those using selective lysis two use aperture impedance signals as the end point while one uses optical scatter. Of the two using granule structure one uses low angle scatter and polarization (Abbott) while the other uses scatter with aperture impedance (Coulter).

RETICULOCYTES

The most recent addition to the multiparameter cell counters are methods to count reticulocytes as a percentage of RBCs. TOA was the first to introduce a reticulocyte counter for the clinical laboratory which uses a fluorescent stain (auramine-O) detected by fluorescence flow cytometry in a separate analyzer. At the present time four methods have been introduced. They use different stains and different means of detection. Coulter and Abbott use the traditional new methylene blue stain. Coulter detects and counts the reticulocytes in the VCS cell

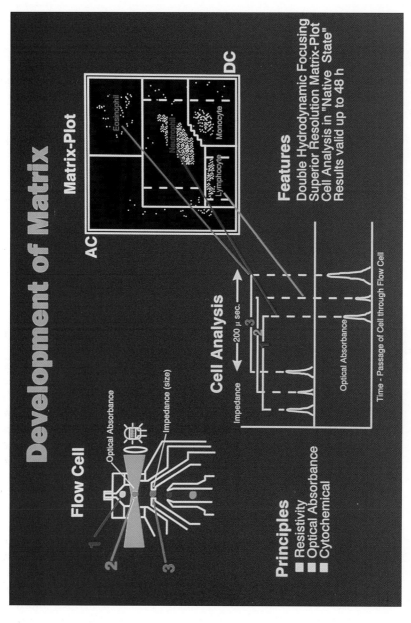

Plate IX Development of the white blood cell classification matrix used on the Roche five part differential systems. Courtesy of Roche Diagnostics, Branchburg, NJ, USA

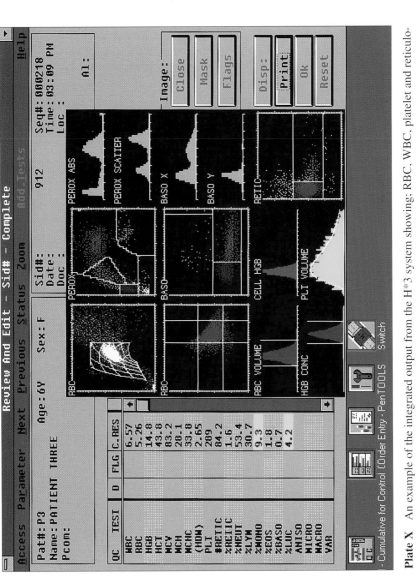

Plate X An example of the integrated output from the H*3 system showing: RBC, WBC, platelet and reticulocyte classification. Courtesy of Bayer Diagnostics, Tarreytown, NY, USA

counter while Abbott uses the MAPSS technology. Bayer uses the optical absorption of an Oxazine-750 dye in the helium neon laser channel of the Technicon H*3 analyzers. In the Bayer system reticulocytes are measured while the RBC are sphered as in the Bayer RBC method. Thus, the reticulocytes may be integrated into the distributions of RBC volume and hemoglobin content. Plate X shows the output of the Bayer No. 3 system including the reticulocyte count.

REFERENCES

Jackson, S.R. and Carter, J.M. (1993) Platelet volume: laboratory measurement and clinical application. *Blood Reviews* **7**: 104.

Kim, Y.R. and Ornstein, L. (1983) Isovolumetric sphering of erythrocytes for more accurate and precise volume measurement by flow cytometry. *Cytometry* **3**(b): 419.

Chapter 4

Standardization

INTRODUCTION/DEFINITIONS

In this chapter we will consider the subject of standardizing the results obtained with multiparameter cell counters; that is, the elimination of biases in the analytical process.

As an illustration consider that initially (day 1) a person's blood is analyzed in New York City on a Technicon H*3. The person then travels to Europe and at the end of a week (day 8), a new specimen is drawn and analyzed in London on a Coulter MAXM system. The following week the same person travels to Asia and a third specimen is drawn and analyzed on day 14 in Tokyo on a Sysmex NE-8000 system. On day 20 the blood from the same person is again drawn and analyzed in San Francisco on an Abbott CD-3000 system, on day 25 blood is drawn and analyzed in Houston on a Roche ARGOS and on day 30 after the person returns to New York City once again the blood is drawn and analyzed on the same Technicon H*3 analyzer. Ideally, we would expect that any changes observed in the hemoglobin or cell counts as the person travelled around the world were the results of biological variations and not due to the fact that the analysis was performed at a different time, a different place, or that a different instrument was used for the analysis. It is by the process of standardization that we expect to reach this ideal.

There are two procedures which are used as part of the standardization process to eliminate analytical biases: *calibration* by which we adjust an instrument to eliminate a bias and *quality control* by which we assure that the instrument remains correctly calibrated. More precise definitions regarding these procedures and the materials used have been published by the International Committee for Standardization in Hematology (ICSH) (Van Assendelft and England, 1982) and the NCCLS and are being developed by the National Reference System for

Practical Guide to Modern Hematology Analyzers. W. Groner and E. Simson
© 1995 John Wiley & Sons Ltd

the Clinical Laboratory. The following definitions are abstracted from those published by the ICSH:

1. *Calibration of the analyzer.* Calibration is the determination of a bias conversion factor of an analytic process under specified conditions in order to obtain accurate measurement results. The accuracy over the operating range is established by appropriate use of reference methods, reference materials, and/or calibrators. Calibration may be performed initially at the manufacturing site, on installation or periodically as indicated by the manufacturer.
2. *Quality control of the analyzer.* Quality control is the set of procedures used to ensure that the instrument is performing over its operating range and that all biases since it was calibrated due to drift or imprecision are within a pre-selected range (the control range). The quality control procedures are used to determine whether the instrument requires recalibration.
3. *Reference method.* A clearly and exactly described technique for a particular determination that will, in the opinion of a competent authority, provide sufficiently accurate and precise laboratory results for this determination. The accuracy of the reference method must be established by comparison with a definitive method where one exists and must be stated. The degree of imprecision of the reference method must also be specified.
4. *Reference material.* A substance or physical device, one or more properties of which have been defined by a definitive or reference method. It is to be used for the verification of the accuracy of an analytical process (measurement system) used in routine practice. Reference materials should be based on or traceable to a national certified reference material or an international (certified) reference preparation.
5. *Selected method.* A procedure, the reliability of which has been validated by a collaborative study and is recommended by a competent authority for use in laboratory analysis. It has been selected on the grounds of its accuracy, precision, economy and ease of performance.
6. *Calibrator.* The ICSH defines a calibrator as: "A substance or device used to calibrate, graduate or adjust a measurement. It must be traceable to a reference standard".
7. *Quality control material.* A substance used in routine practice for checking the concurrent performance of an analytical process (or instrument). It must be similar in properties to and analyzed along with patient specimens. It should preferably have a pre-assigned value.

In considering the practical application of these definitions to the problems of standardizing the hematology analyzer results in the illustration given above it is quickly apparent that there are three tacit assumptions which are also made:

- That there is an internationally accepted and easily practiced reference method for each of the parameters in the complete blood count and WBC differential.
- That it is practical to compare the results obtained on blood specimens between a cell counting instrument and the reference methods.
- That there exists a means by which the instrument can be adjusted to eliminate bias between its results and those obtained with the reference method or by use of a reference material.

It will be seen in the following sections that these assumptions are not appropriate for all of the parameters which are reported on modern cell counters. Thus the problem of standardization of modern hematology analyzers remains very much an open issue. In the remainder of this chapter we will discuss the applications of the concepts of standardization defined above to modern cell counters and indicate the current status and open issues.

We will consider first the problems of calibration of the instrument, and then consider quality control. Finally, we will turn to the most difficult problem of all "setting performance goals" for the modern cell counters. In setting performance goals for hematology analyzers one must estimate what degree of standardization is desirable and necessary for various clinical purposes recognizing that perfect standardization is probably an unattainable ideal.

CALIBRATION

The calibration of a modern multiparameter hematology instrument involves adjustments to correct for the dilution factor and signal amplitude in each of the channels. From the system descriptions given in Chapter 3 it is seen that this requires adjustment of the biases with regard to a minimum of six different hematological parameters:

1. The white blood cell count.
2. The red blood cell count.
3. The packed cell volume or the MCV.
4. The hemoglobin concentration.
5. The platelet count.
6. The sub-classifications of white blood cells (WBC differential).

These adjustments may be made either by comparing the values recovered by the instrument on fresh whole blood with values obtained by a reference method, or through the use of intermediary materials, i.e.

Table 4.1 Status of reference method development for hematology parameters

Parameter	ICSH	NCCLS	Issues
Hemoglobin	Published. HiCN international ref. material	Approved H15. HiCN	Filtration to eliminate turbidity from RBC stroma
Packed cell volume	Published. Macro-crit corrected for plasma trapping	Approved H7. Micro-crit uncorrected for plasma trapping	Plasma trapping
WBC count	Published (ZBI method)		
RBC count	Published (ZBI method)		
Platelet count	In development (indirect platelet count by flow cytometry)		Direct vs indirect
WBC differential	In development Flow cytometry	Approved H20. Microscopic method 400 cells. Romanowsky stain	Precision
Cell size analysis	Published (log normal fitting)		Log normal for RBC
Mean cell volume (RBC)	In development		
Reticulocyte count	In development (visual ratio count)	In development (fluorescent flow cytometer ratio count)	Visual vs flow

calibrators such as stabilized blood whose recovery relative to whole blood is known and to which a proper calibration value has been assigned. In either case, it is first necessary to have a procedure with which to establish reference values for each of the parameters to be calibrated on whole blood specimens. This is done by use of a reference material and/or a reference method. Reference methods and materials are typically developed by the committees of Standards Organizations such as the ICSH or the NCCLS which comprise laboratory scientists as well as representatives from the manufacturers of cell counters.

Table 4.1 summarizes the status of the pertinent reference methods for hematology. It can be seen that for some hematology parameters there is more than one reference method while for others there is no reference method or the reference method is currently being developed. It is also seen that in some cases (notably the packed cell volume) there may be some differences between the reference methods adopted by the different organizations. This could result in a bias between instruments whose calibration is referred to different reference methods. Fortunately these differences are small and mainly of academic interest. It can also be seen in Table 4.1 that at present there are five items on the list of six parameters above for which an accepted reference method or material exists. The following briefly describes the accepted reference methods.

1. *The total hemoglobin concentration* (ICSH, 1978). Both the NCCLS and ICSH reference methods are based on the absorption of light after the red blood cells are lysed and the hemoglobin converted to cyanmethemoglobin (HiCN).
2. *The packed cell volume* (ICSH, 1980). The ICSH reference method employs a Wintrobe tube and a correction for the plasma trapped when the blood is packed. The NCCLS uses a micro-crit tube without a correction for trapped plasma. Since plasma trapping in the smaller diameter tube is smaller and is also counterbalanced by red cell dehydration, only a small difference (approximately 1%) exists between the methods.
3. *The WBC differential* (NCCLS, 1992). The reference method for the leukocyte differential has been established by the NCCLS and published in document H20-A. It involves the microscopic analysis of 400 white blood cells after staining with Romanowsky stains.
4. *Red cell count* (ICSH, 1994). The reference method for the red cell count specifies a semi-automated blood cell counter in which the particle count can be determined for a fixed and known fluid volume (the procedure utilizes the Coulter ZBI which is an electronic cell counter that meets this criterion). Two sequential dilutions are made into isotonic buffered saline for a total of 1/50 000. Coincidence is measured and corrected.
   - 1/amplification = 1.
   - 1/aperture current = 0.34.
   - Counting volume (validated by manufacturer) = 0.4 (typically 0.0025 ml).

   The results are corrected for coincidence and dilution using the chart provided by the manufacturer, but since the chart assumes a dilution of 50 000, the resulting answer has to be multiplied by 50 601/50 000.
5. *White cell count* (ICSH, 1994). This count also may be performed with the Coulter ZBI under the same counting conditions. However, only the first dilution is used and the count performed 1 to 5 minutes after the addition of Zap-oglobin (Coulter electronics). For

the platelet count in the absence of a reference method the ICSH has published guidelines for selected methods to be used in calibrating or assigning values to calibrators. The ICSH selected methods, which appear below, follow the procedures described by Rowan (1988).

6. *Platelet count*. The selected method for platelet counting is by hemocytometry. The counting chambers (hemocytometers) should be of the Neubauer design and have an inaccuracy of the specified volume of less than 1%. The diluting fluid should be 1% ammonium oxalate prepared from analytical grade reagant dissolved in deionized water and filtered through a 0.22 μm membrane filter and stored at 4°C. All glassware used should be certified: less than 1% for small volumes and grade A for large volumes. The blood specimens should be anticoagulated with EDTA at 1.5–2.0 mg/ml and should be no more than 4 hours old when analyzed: 2 dilutions (1:20) of freshly mixed blood in ammonium oxalate solution should be prepared and mixed for 10 minutes. Each dilution should be used to fill two counting chambers, and then left to settle in a moist atmosphere for 2.0 minutes. The chambers should then be counted with a phase contrast microscope. The accuracy of this method is limited by the number of cells counted. For a total of 500 platelets, the coefficient variation will be 5%; thus, for a platelet count of 150×10^9 per liter, the 95% confidence limits within which the true results may lie will be from 135×10^9 per liter to 165×10^9 per liter.

7. *Indirect platelet count*. An alternative selected method which is recommended by the ICSH for obtaining the platelet count is the automated indirect platelet count obtained by using an instrument which accurately determines the ratio of platelets to red blood cells for a minimum of 50 000 cells. The resulting ratio may then be multiplied by the red blood cell count obtained with the reference method described above to obtain the platelet count.

INSTRUMENT CALIBRATION PROCEDURES

Calibration of a modern hematology analyzer typically involves two distinct steps: in the first step the instrument is standardized; and in the second step the instrument is adjusted to eliminate any biases between the values produced and those of the reference or selected method. The procedure for standardization is instrument specific and is generally described in the user's manual. It consists of a series of checks and adjustments which must be made to insure that the instrument is in good working condition and all adjustments (such as thresholds and electronic gains) and alignments (optical or mechanical) are in their nominal positions. Failure to complete this step before actually running a calibrator on the system can lead to errors in accuracy which are not easily detected. For instance, a misplaced discriminator threshold for counting may eliminate from the post detection algorithm some fraction of the calibrator cells. This can lead to an error in calibration if there is not an exact overlap in the signal amplitude histogram between the cells of whole blood specimens and those of the calibrant.

Once the system has been standardized, the actual calibration can take place by analyzing the sample to which measured values have been previously assigned and adjusting the analyzer's post-detection algorithm, to recover these preassigned values. Materials which are used in the process may take one of two forms: fresh whole blood; or stabilized blood and/or other surrogate materials. The following paragraphs briefly describe the nature and use of each type of material.

Fresh whole blood

In calibration with fresh whole blood, the blood specimens are used as a medium to transfer the reference values obtained using the reference or selected methods indicated above to the instrument to be calibrated. Of particular concern in this procedure is the freshness of the sample i.e. the procedure must be completed before any changes in the whole blood specimen have occurred due to aging. Sufficient numbers of whole blood specimens must be used to overcome any random variation between the reference methods and the instrument to be calibrated. For example, assume that it is desired to calibrate the results to an accuracy of 1% and the random variation between the instrument method and the reference method is known to be 2%. Then it is necessary to average the bias results obtained from at least four different specimens in order to calculate the correct bias conversion factor. This procedure is outlined in schematic form in Figure 4.1, while Table 4.2 shows the number of blood samples which are required to achieve a stipulated calibration accuracy (Groner, 1982). The specimen characteristics which are required to avoid interferences are also listed in the table.

Stabilized blood or surrogate materials

In this procedure the specimen is a stabilized whole blood specimen or other surrogate material for which values for calibration have been preassigned. It is assumed that these values are stable between the time of assignment and the time of use. The procedure for value assignment of a stabilized blood specimen involves the determination of recovery ratios between the stabilized material and fresh whole blood whose values have been established by the use of reference and/or selected

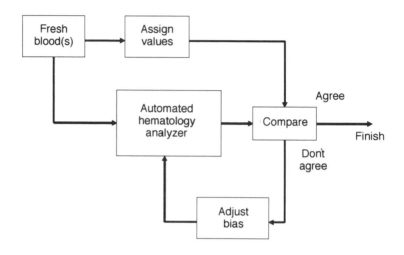

Figure 4.1   Calibration by transfer from whole blood

Table 4.2   Whole blood calibration: minimum numbers and characteristics of normal specimens required to calibrate to a desired accuracy

Parameter	Desired accuracy (%)	Number of specimens	Characteristics
Red blood count	1	5	RBC between
	2	2	2000×10^9 and
	3	1	6000×10^9
White blood count	2	11	WBC between
	4	3	3.0×10^9 and
			40×10^9
Packed cell	2	10	Oxygenate fully
volume	3	5	MCHC normal
	4	3	MCV normal
Hemoglobin	1	7	WBC less than
	2	2	40×10^9
	3	1	
Platelet count	2	15	MPV greater than
	4	4	5.5 fl
	6	2	

Table 4.3 Value assignment methods used by some manufacturers of calibrators for multiparameter cell counters

Parameter	ICSH method	Coulter	Bayer	Roche	Streck	R & D systems
RBC count	ZBI	ZBI	ZBI	ZBI	ZBI	ZBI
WBC count	ZBI	ZBI	ZBI	ZBI	ZBI	ZBI
Hb	ICSH HiCN	NCCLS H15	NCCLS H15	NCCLS H15	NCCLS H15	NCCLS H15
PCV	Macro or micro	NCCLS H7	NCCLS H7	NCCLS H7	NCCLS H7	NCCLS H7
WBC differential	NCCLS H20	NCCLS H20		Visual	—	—
Platelet	Phase or indirect	Phase	Phase	Phase	Phase	Phase
MCV	Derived	Derived	Derived	Derived	Derived	Derived
RDW	—	—	—	—	—	—
MPV	—	Latex	—	—	—	—

methods. The values are then assigned to the calibrator using the simple formula:

$$Value\ (assigned) = \frac{V_{cal}}{V_{blood}}\ Ref_{blood}$$

Where V_{cal} and V_{blood} are the values recovered for the calibrator and whole blood respectively and Ref_{blood} is the reference value for the whole blood.

This is typically performed in the manufacturer's laboratory using the average from a sufficient number of whole blood specimens to assure accuracy. Thus, the single assigned value may be used in calibration by the user laboratory. Table 4.3 gives the reference methods used by the manufacturers of modern cell counters in assigning reference values to whole blood specimens.

CALIBRATION OF THE WBC DIFFERENTIAL

Calibration of the WBC differential presents a unique problem. Although a reference method exists, there is generally no means by which the instrument recovery can be adjusted to correct a bias by the user. The algorithms and measurements by which the cells are classified are essentially determined at manufacture and remain an intrinsic part of the instrument. The algorithms and measurements are sensitive to signal amplitude. Therefore instrument standardization procedures are important to their proper function. However, for these parameters the calibration procedure ends with instrument standardization.

QUALITY CONTROL

The purpose of quality control (QC) is to ensure that that the analyzer continues to perform with the expected precision and linearity and has not drifted from the time that calibration was performed. This is done by monitoring results obtained within the laboratory (intralaboratory QC) and/or by comparing results obtained in the laboratory to those obtained on the same specimen in other laboratories (interlaboratory QC).

INTRALABORATORY QUALITY CONTROL

Methods of intralaboratory quality control as practiced in other laboratories like the clinical chemistry laboratory typically rely on "truth in a bottle" and involve the repeated sampling of a specimen containing purified weighed-in material standards. However, with automated multiparameter cell counters, this straightforward approach is not feasible because of the complex nature of the hematology analytes and the lability of the hematology sample. With the exception of the single analyte hemoglobin, it is not possible to prepare, transport, and preserve standards containing reference values for the cell counting parameters. To circumvent these deficiencies a number of quality control strategies have evolved. These can be characterized in terms of the materials used:

- Fresh blood (repeated sampling).
- Commercial controls (stabilized human or animal blood).
- Statistical functions of patient measurements (moving averages).

Because no single approach is ideal, it is not surprising that in addition to the use of one of these techniques various permutations and combinations of the above methods have also been suggested and used. In the following paragraphs we will discuss the application of these techniques to modern hematology analyzers:

1. Monitoring drift.
2. Determining imprecision.
3. Determining nonlinearity.

Monitoring drift

To insure accurate results it is necessary periodically to verify the instrument's calibration. This is done conceptually by repeated analysis of the same specimens which are assumed to be stable over a significant time interval. However, the stability of fresh whole blood is extremely limited; hence the simple procedure of holding a blood specimen for repeated analysis for periods greater than 4 or 6 hours is fraught with the difficulty of determining whether the observed changes are due to changes in the specimen or drift in the instrument. Two means have been employed to overcome this difficulty and allow the monitoring of more stable materials to assure the constancy of calibration over extended periods:

1. The use of stabilized blood as a control material.
2. The use of certain average values obtained in processing whole blood specimens that have been found to be relatively constant.

The use of stabilized blood as a quality control material

Stabilized blood controls are manufactured from human or animal blood cells which are preserved in a special plasma replacement fluid. Depending upon the manufacturer, the cells may have been treated with a stabilizing agent or lightly fixed with a chemical cross-linker like formaldehyde before resuspension. In general the dating of these materials is limited to less than two months. During this period the controls are analyzed periodically on the instrument along with patient specimens, and their value is recorded at each analysis to compare with the previous values. The stabilized controls usually have preassigned values. The control range, i.e. the range accepted for recovery at any given sampling of the stabilized controls, is determined by the precision of the instrument, the stability of the material, and the strategy (frequency) of use. Manufacturers generally supply the material, together with a recommended control range. In this case, the stated control range is equal to the range beyond which there is a 95% chance of instrument drift on a single determination. Table 4.4 summarizes the control ranges given by the manufacturers of modern cell counters based on the coefficient of variation (CV) of the recovery. Note that the 95% control range is equivalent to two times the CV.

As in the recovery of any specimen the effects of imprecision can be reduced by the reciprocal of the square root of N, where N is the number of samplings. Thus, the more often a control is sampled the more precisely the actual recovery is known and as a consequence the smaller the amount of drift that it is possible to detect. Many different

Table 4.4 Typical control ranges (2CV) for hematology parameters from manufacturers of multiparameter cell counters

Parameter	Level	Coulter (%)	Bayer (%)	TOA (%)	Roche (%)	Abbott (%)
RBC	Low	5.0	6.5	5.0	4.5	3.5
RBC	Normal	3.0	4.5	4.5	3.5	3.5
Hemoglobin	Low	6.0	5.0	5.0	6.0	4.5
Hemoglobin	Normal	3.0	3.0	4.0	3.5	3.0
PCV	Low	10.0	6.0	6.5	11.0	6.7
PCV	Normal	4.5	6.0	6.0	5.0	3.8
MCV	Normal	3.5	5.5	4.5	3.8	2.0
MCH	Normal	4.0	5.0	5.0	6.5	5.0
MCHC	Normal	5.0	6.5	6.0	8.0	8.0
RDW	Normal	11.0	17.0	—	19.0	14.5
Platelet	Low	18.0	20.0	24.0	30.0	14.0
Platelet	Normal	10.0	13.0	14.0	10.0	14.0
MPV	Normal	20.0	14.0	—	25.0	14.0
WBC count	Low	14.0	8.5	17.0	12.0	17.0
WBC count	Normal	6.5	9.2	11.0	6.5	13.0
WBC count	High	17.05	13.0	10.0	5.0	6.5
Neuts (%)	Normal	10.0	15.0	8.0	8.0	8.0
Lymphs (%)	Normal	20.0	22.0	20.0	16.0	13.0
Mono (%)	Normal	23.0	72.0	61.0	37.0	—
Eos (%)	Normal	50.0	100.0	37.0	50.0	—
Baso (%)	Normal	200	100.0	—	50.0	—

strategies for sampling the control material are employed. In general, they attempt to optimize the quality of results, by balancing the tightness of control range on the one hand against the cost of the quality control material on the other hand.

The use of moving averages

Laboratories which analyze a large number of samples have an alternative means to monitor drift in instrument calibration for some measurements. This is accomplished by observing trends in the average value of certain parameters over a large number of patient samples. It has been demonstrated (Bull *et al.*, 1974) that certain parameters of patient specimens such as the mean red cell hemoglobin concentration are geographically invariant (same mean value all over the earth) and vary over a relatively narrow range in both health and disease. Thus, the tracking of averages of these values provides an alternative for monitoring drift. In this application the average value of the patient specimens is treated as the equivalent to a stable quality control material and is tracked using a moving average algorithm (Korpman and Bull, 1976).

Optimization is a tradeoff between the sensitivity of detection (narrow control range) and the speed of response (number of samples averaged) (Bull, 1984).

For most practical applications, the only parameters in the modern CBC instruments which have sufficiently narrow biological variation to be used in such a scheme are the red cell indices (MCV, MCH and MCHC), especially MCHC and MCH and to a much lesser extent, MCV. However, investigations are continuing regarding the ratio of other parameters such as the red blood cell count divided by the platelet count as well as the ratio of some elements of the WBC differential.

Monitoring imprecision

The reproducibility or precision of the instrument is a major factor in instrument performance. However, it is generally measured indirectly by determining the imprecision or the differences in results which result from the lack of reproducibility of the instrument.

The difference between two sequential patient results cannot be compared for clinical purposes with finer resolution than that given by the imprecision of the instrument. Specifically, if the difference between two sequential test results obtained from separate specimens is less then 1.4 times the coefficient of variation obtained by running repeated results on the first specimen, then there is a high probability (37%) that the true patient's values are, in fact, identical.

In cell counters one fundamental source of imprecision is given by the number of particles in the sample analyzed. The frequency distribution for the number of particles (μ) actually encountered in repeated sampling of a specimen which contains an average number (n) particles per unit volume has been shown to be:

$$P(\mu) = \frac{e^n n^\mu}{\mu!}$$

This distribution is generally called the Poisson distribution. Although, it is different from the more familiar normal distribution, it shares the property that for large n the variance is equal to the mean. As a result, for particle counting the coefficient of variation (CV) is given simply by:

$$CV = \frac{\text{Variance}}{\text{Mean}} = \frac{1}{\sqrt{n}}$$

Thus, the minimum difference in cell counts which can be detected between two successive counts on the same specimen, even with a perfect cell counter, is proportional to the reciprocal of the square root of the average number of cells which are counted. It was noted in the previous chapter that most modern cell counters count approximately the number of red blood cells contained in 0.01 μl of blood, count the platelets along with the red cells, and count approximately the number of white blood cells contained in 1 μl of the original specimen. Using the equation above we can estimate the fundamental imprecision of sampling for a normal specimen with 5 million RBCs per μl, 20/1 ratio of RBCs to platelets, and a 7500 per μl WBC count, i.e.

$$CV \ (RBC) = 0.45\%$$
$$CV \ (platelet) = 2.0 \ \%$$
$$CV \ (WBC) = 1.1\%$$

It is seen that, except for platelets, the statistical sampling error is less than or equal to the precision of dilution which is typically around 1% (see Chapter 2). Typical values for the imprecision of multiparameter cell counters are given in terms of the coefficient of variation obtained by running repeated results. They are generally somewhat greater than that given by the sampling imprecision alone and except for platelets show the effects of the imprecision of dilution.

The imprecision of cell sizing results is generally smaller than those obtained for the cell counts. This is because the results are generally obtained by averaging over a substantial number of size signals, and since the cell size distribution is an intrinsic factor of the specimen there is no variation in results due to the imprecision of dilution.

Determining nonlinearity

Cell counting

The implicit assumptions which were made in calibrating the instrument by recovering the assigned value of the calibrator are that the instrument responds only to particles and that there is a linear relationship between particle concentration and the resulting cell count. Thus, when the particle density goes to zero, the count should also go to zero. The cell counting process, however (as explained in Chapter 2), is intrinsically linear only over a restricted range of counts. At sufficiently high counts there is a growing probability of coincidence (two or more cells will be in the sensing zone at the same time) resulting in underrecovery compared to a linear extrapolation. Further, at extremely low cell counts there will be added counts due to background counts (spurious signals caused by electronic noise) leading to overrecovery compared to a linear extrapolation. Imprecision will also increase at low levels, i.e. precision will get worse, due to increasing statistical variation of the small number of cells counted. Thus, in general, both error due to the nonlinearity of the cell counter and the background count can be a source of nonlinearity at low counts.

The required range of values over which cell counters must perform is determined by the variation in the specimens. This may be substantial. Therefore, maintaining the standardization of the counter over the assay range must encompass verification of the linearity. There are two ways to accomplish this:

1. The use of stabilized blood at different concentration levels.
2. Dilution experiments.

In the first method, stabilized blood is prepared at different concentrations (typically 2 or 3), and a measured value assigned to each. The materials are then re-assayed periodically and the results are compared to the previously assigned value.

In the second approach, a concentrated sample is made from fresh whole blood and then carefully diluted down serially. Correct dilution can be a particularly difficult problem in hematology where the specimen is a non-Newtonian two phase fluid. Consequently, errors in dilution are quite easy to make. One means of avoiding this type of error is to verify each dilution by making a reference assay such as the total hemoglobin.

Cell size

Monitoring the linearity of cell size determinations in a quality control program presents a more difficult problem and is essentially intractable for modern cell counters. It is not possible to vary the cell size through dilution experiments, nor is it possible to maintain stable standards at various cell sizes. Thus, the monitoring of linearity for the cell size parameters is generally accomplished by repeated analysis of a stabilized blood preparation. However, the process of stabilization generally involves changes in the physical properties of the blood cells which are then detected differently by the different detection systems (see Chapter 2). Thus, the recovered values for the same stabilized materials obtained on different cell counting systems may be quite different even when the systems give the same results on fresh whole blood specimens.

The WBC differential

Quality control of the WBC differential raises several problems, some of which were addressed above in discussing calibration of the WBC differential. In addition, because of the different technologies used by different analyzers for classifying leukocytes, it is extremely difficult to provide a stabilized blood preparation which will be suitable for more than one make of analyzer.

INTERLABORATORY QUALITY ASSESSMENT

The second means for monitoring the performance of hematology analyzers is by the use of external quality assessment. In this technique, the state of the calibration of an analyzer is verified by comparing the results obtained on the same samples with those obtained on a large number of instruments, each of which is independently standardized, calibrated, and quality controlled. Unfortunately, this technique is also fundamentally limited by the availability of a fresh blood sample. Thus, if one uses a fresh unstabilized sample the test is limited by the logistics of sample handling and sample transport. On the other hand, if a stabilized blood is employed, the test result may be suspect due to the unknown differences in physical properties between the test specimen and fresh whole blood which may affect the recovered results. The effects resulting from the difference between the sample and typical specimens are generally called matrix effects. Matrix effects on the measurement are especially apparent when the test specimen is analyzed using counters which employ different counting and sizing technology. For instance, the technique of stabilizing red blood cells by fixation with a cross-linking agent will affect the index of a fraction, the dielectrical permeability of the membrane, and the cell deformability. Optical cell counters may react to the changes in refractive index while aperture impedance counters react to the changes in dielectric and deformability properties. Two different instruments which have been carefully calibrated to give similar results for MCV on fresh whole blood specimens may thus give quite different results on such a stabilized test specimen. In the particular case of MCV, the variation and mean value between the different classes of instrument generally reported in interlaboratory quality control summaries may reflect only the properties of the specimen and not analyzer performance.

A similar situation exists for the components of the WBC differential where the methods of preserving the leukocytes, in general, affect the parameters which are measured (size, granularity, etc.). As with the red blood cells the different measurement methods are affected differently. For this reason interlaboratory quality control results for the WBC differential can only be considered valid within a single instrument class and results are usually tabulated in this way.

In the results of interlaboratory quality control data, a second source of error due to the specimen arises from the fact that the stabilized material may not respond to all elements of the measurement process.

For instance, quality control specimens consisting of partially fixed red blood cells or surrogate white blood cells may not demonstrate the same variation in the selective lytic processes which are used within the instrument to discriminate cell types as would a fresh whole blood cell sample. Thus, they may not truly represent the status of the instrument regarding fresh blood specimens.

In spite of the cautions listed above, the results of interlaboratory quality assessment trials provide substantial data regarding the standardization of the results of multiparameter cell counting instruments. Participation in external quality assessment programs (run either by national organizations or by manufacturers) is generally available for the traditional CBC parameters. Results, typically, indicate the laboratory's performance relative to a peer group. In addition, summary results are published periodically in the literature. The situation for the WBC differential, however, is much different. Only limited programs are available. Further, these programs use different materials (specimens) tailored to each of the specific instrument classes. Thus, it is not possible to compare results for the automated WBC differential even on stabilized material across the instruments of different manufacturers.

PERFORMANCE GOALS FOR CELL COUNTERS

The purpose of a quality assurance program is to ensure that the results of an analytic method live up to a set of predetermined ideals. Therefore, goals for analytic performance need to be defined. The more specific the definition is, the more focused the quality assurance program can be. In addition to providing an objective against which to measure whether or not acceptable quality is being achieved, explicit performance goals are integral to the design of the QC program. That is, they indicate what to monitor and with what accuracy.

Traditionally, in the clinical laboratory desired performance is firmly anchored in the physical and/or chemical standards (i.e. the truth in the bottle concept). Further, for many of the serum analytes reference methods which may be practically used to determine bias exist. Also interlaboratory trials are available giving consensus results on standard materials. Thus, for most of the analytes in the serum chemistry laboratory standards for performance can be set in terms of bias and imprecision with regard to recovering "truth". However, even for these analytes a more complex problem is relating the determination of performance achieved to the clinician's need. That is, even when we can easily determine how good a measurement is, we are still faced with the problem of stating how good it should be so as to estimate whether it is "good enough" for clinical use.

Two basic approaches have been used to set analytic goals for the variability of results from a laboratory determination; the questionnaire and consensus. In the questionnaire method a large number of physicians are asked how large a change in the result would be considered medically significant (i.e. requiring action) at or near the medical decision level. For example, would further clinical study be prompted by a change of hemoglobin of 0.1 g at 11.0 g, or if not, would a change of 0.2 g stimulate action. In the second approach the standard for performance is derived from the consensus of results obtained on a specimen as in a interlaboratory trial. That is, if 95% of the determinations for hemoglobin on a single sample of reference material made at different laboratories vary by 0.2 g then the performance ideal for any laboratory is to maintain variability to less than 0.2 g.

Both of these approaches are unsatisfactory, in that they tend to emphasize the status quo. The true clinical value of reduced variability could not be assessed by physicians who have no experience with this level of precision. Thus, the tendency in questionnaire responses is to reflect what the physicians are accustomed to or the current state of the art. Similarly, consensus merely establishes the state of the current art, without regard to clinical need.

In order to find an approach which avoids subjectivity, a group of clinical chemists, pathologists, statisticians, and other laboratory scientists met in Aspen, Colorado, USA, in 1976 to discuss ways to set analytic goals for the clinical laboratory. They reached a tentative consensus which was set forth in their report, "Analytical Goals in Clinical Chemistry" (Elevitch, 1976) which was subsequently approved by the Subcommittee on Analytic Goals in Clinical Chemistry of the World Association of Societies of Pathology. The chief recommendations of this report were:

1. Analytical goals can only be defined in terms of the needs for patient care. Any other basis is irrelevant.
2. Goals for precision and accuracy of quantitative methods, where the analytes are well defined, should be at least as stringent as the current performance by well-managed laboratories, or the state of the art.
3. For group screening, in which an individual is to be selected from a population, a goal for analytic coefficient of variation is defined as:

$$CV_a \leqslant 1/2\sqrt{CV^2_{intra} + CV^2_{norm}}$$

Where the CV_{intra} and the CV_{norm} are the intraindividual and interindividual biologic variations respectively.

4. For testing to evaluate a diagnosis or monitor treatment of an individual, a goal for analytic coefficient of variation is defined as:

$$CV_a \leqslant 1/2 \ CV_{intra}$$

5. There is a major need for further study and understanding of statistical relationships that should be used to derive a clinical diagnosis from an analytical value.

6. When the physiological and pathophysiological mechanisms which produce biologic variations are understood, it may be possible to reduce the effects of the biologic variation on total observed variability.

Thus, in summary, the group of scientists established another means for setting goals for the variability in analytic performance by comparing it to biologic variation. The Subcommittee on Quantitative Cellular Hematology of the NCCLS has tried to apply this principle to cell counting in the hematology laboratory in their proposed document H26-P "Performance Goals for the Internal Quality Control of Multichannel Hematology Analyzers" (NCCLS, 1989). This document sets forth the goals for some of the hematology parameters. Table 4.5 gives the proposed standards for bias, precision and total variability as stated in H26 for five common parameters.

Table 4.5 Performance goals (%) for hematology parameters (adapted from H26)

Parameter	Level	Bias goal (2CV)	Precision (CV)	Total (2CV)
WBC count	$1.0 \times 10^9/l$	9.8	8.0	12.7
WBC count	$6.0 \times 10^9/l$	9.8	8.0	12.7
WBC count	$20.0 \times 10^9/l$	9.8	8.0	12.7
RBC count	$2.7 \times 10^{12}/l$	3.9	3.2	5.1
RBC count	$4.7 \times 10^{12}/l$	3.4	2.5	4.2
RBC count	$6.6 \times 10^{12}/l$	3.5	2.5	4.3
Hemoglobin	8.0 g/dl	4.3	4.5	6.3
Hemoglobin	14.0 g/dl	3.1	2.0	3.7
Hemoglobin	20.0 g/dl	3.7	2.8	4.6
MCV	60 fl	3.3	2.8	4.3
MCV	90 lf	2.8	2.2	3.6
MCV	120 fl	2.9	2.3	3.7
Platelets	$50 \times 10^9/l$	14.7	9.9	17.7
Platelets	$300 \times 10^9/l$	14.7	9.9	17.7
Platelets	$800 \times 10^9/l$	14.7	9.9	17.7

Table 4.6 Performance goals vs control ranges for multiparameter cell counters

Parameter	Level	Performance goal total from Table 4.5 (%)	Average manufacturer control range (%)
RBC count	Low	5.1	4.9
RBC count	Normal	4.2	3.8
Hemoglobin	Low	6.3	5.3
Hemoglobin	Normal	3.7	3.3
WBC count	Low	12.7	13.7
WBC count	Normal	12.7	9.2
WBC count	High	12.7	8.3
Platelet	Low	17.7	21.0
Platelet	Normal	17.7	12.2
MCV	Normal	3.6	3.8

It is interesting to compare the performance standards given in the proposed NCCLS document to the control ranges recommended by the manufacturers of multiparameter cell counters. Table 4.6 makes this comparison. For most of the traditional hematology parameters the control ranges are close to the standards set in H26-P. However, similar analysis for the new hematology parameters (WBC differential, and size parameters) has not yet been established. We will be talking a great deal more about this in the next chapter when we consider the performance of the modern multiparameter cell counters.

REFERENCES

Bull, B.S. (1984) Quality assurance strategies. In Koepke, J. (ed.) *Laboratory Hematology*, pp. 999–1023. Churchill-Livingstone, Edinburgh and London.
Bull, B.S., Elashoff, R.M., Heilbron, D.C. and Couperus, J. (1974) A study of various estimators for the derivation of quality control procedures from patient erythrocyte indices. *Am. J. Clin. Pathol.* **61**: 473–81.
Elevitch. Fr (ed.) (1976) College of American Pathologists Conference Report. Conference on Analytical Goals in Clinical Chemistry, at Aspen CO. Skokie IL, CAP.
Groner, W. (1982) Specification of calibration, control and reference materials for cell counting and sizing apparatus. In Van Assendelft, O.W. and England, J.M. (eds.) *Advances in Hematological Methods: The Blood Count*, pp. 185–95. CRC Press, Boca Raton, FL.
ICSH (1978) Recommendations for reference method for haemoglobinometry in human blood and specifications for international haemoglobincyanide reference preparation. *J. Clin. Pathol.* **31**: 139–43.

ICSH (1980) Recommendation for reference method for determination by centrifugation of packed cell volume of blood. *J. Clin. Pathol.* **33**: 1–2.

ICSH (1994) Reference method for the enumeration of erythrocytes and leucocytes. *Clin. Lab. Haemat.* **16**: 131–138.

Korpman, R.A. and Bull, B.S. (1976) The implementation of a robust estimator of the mean for quality control on a programmable calculator or a laboratory computer. *Am. J. Clin. Pathol.* **65**: 252–3.

NCCLS (1984a) *Tentative Standard H20-T: Leukocyte Differential Counting.* NCCLS, Villanova, PA 19085, USA.

NCCLS (1984b) *Approved Standard H-15A. Reference Procedure for the Quantitative Determination of Hemoglobin in Blood.* NCCLS, Villanova, PA 19085, USA.

NCCLS (1985) *Approved Standard H-7A. Procedure for Determining Packed Cell Volume by the Microhematocrit Method.* NCCLS, Villanova, PA 19085, USA.

NCCLS (1989) Proposed Standard H26-P: Performance Goals for the Internal Quality Control of Multichannel Hematology Analyzers 9:(9) NCCLS, Villanova, PA 19085, USA.

Rowan, R.M. (1988) The standardization of calibration and control of instruments and kits. In Lewis, S.M. and Verwilghen, R.L. (eds.) *Quality Assurance in Hematology.* Baillière Tindall, London.

Van Assendelft, O.W. and England, J.M. (1982) Terms, quantities, and units. In van Assendelft, O.W. and England, J.M. (eds.) *Advances in Hematological Methods: the Blood Count*, pp. 1–9. CRC Press, Boca Raton.

FURTHER READING

Berkson, J., Magath, T.B. and Hurn, M. The error of estimate of the blood cell count as made with the hemocytometer. *Am. J. Physiol.*, **128**: 309, 1939.

Broughton, P.M.G., Gowenlock, A.M., McCormack, J.J. and Neill, D.W. (1969) A recommended scheme for the evaluation of instruments for automated analysis in the clinical biochemistry laboratory. *J. Clin. Pathol.* **22**: 278–84.

Broughton, P.M.G., Gowenlock, A.N., McCormak, J.J. and Neill, D.W. (1974) A revised scheme for the evaluation of automated instruments for use in Clinical Chemistry. *Ann. Clin. Biochem.* **11**: 207–13.

England, J.M. (1982) The analysis and interpretation of cell size distribution curves in hematology, a review. In van Assendelft, O.W. and England, J.M. (eds.) *Advances in Hematological Methods: the Blood Count*, pp. 109–123. CRC Press, Boca Raton.

England, J.M. (1986) Internal quality control and calibration. In *Automation and Quality Assurance in Hematology.* Blackwell Scientific Publications.

England, J.M., Chetty, M.C., Garvey, B., Lewis, S.M., Wardle, J., Cousins, S., Crosland-Taylor, P.J. and Syndercombe-Court, D. (1983) Testing of calibration and quality control material use with automatic blood counting apparatus: application of the protocol described by the British Committee of Standardization in Haematology. *Clin. Lab. Haematol.* **5**: 83–92.

Gibson, F.M. (1982) Standardization for routine blood counting. In Cavill, I. (ed.) *Methods in Hematology: Quality Control*, pp. 13–34. Churchill-Livingstone, Edinburgh and London.

Groner, W. (1984) Standardization of multi-parameter instruments for blood cell counting and sizing. In Cavill, I. (ed.) *Methods in Hematology: Quality Control* 2nd edn, pp. 31–54. Churchill-Livingstone, Edinburgh and London.

Helleman, P.W. (1972) Results of a trial on erythrocyte counting. In Izak, G. and Lewis, S.M. (eds.) *Modern Concepts in Hematology*, p. 235. Academic Press, New York.

ICSH (1967) Recommendations for haemiglobinometry in human blood. *Br. J. Haematol.* **13** (Suppl): 71–5.

ICSH (1982) Recommendations for the analysis of red cell, white cell and platelet size distribution curves. I. General Principles. *J. Clin. Pathol.* **35**: 1320–2.

ICSH (1983) Protocol for evaluation of automated blood cell counters. *Clin. Lab. Haematol.* **6**: 69–84.

Koepke, J.A. (1975) Inter-laboratory trials: The quality control survey program of the College of American Pathologists. In Lewis, S.M. and Coster, F.J. (eds.) *Quality Control in Haematology*, pp. 53–67. Academic Press, New York.

NCCLS (1982a) *Tentative Standard H21-T: Standardized Collection, Transport, and Preparation of Blood Specimens for Coagulation Testing.* NCCLS, Villanova, PA 19085, USA.

NCCLS (1982b) *Tentative Guideline EP2-T: Establishing Performance Claims for Clinical Methods, Introduction and Performance Check Experiment.* NCCLS, Villanova, PA 19085, USA.

NCCLS (1982c) *Tentative Guideline EP3-T: Establishing Performance Claims for Clinical Chemical Methods, Replication Experiment.* NCCLS, Villanova, PA 19085, USA.

NCCLS (1982d) *Tentative Guideline EP4-T: Establishing Performance Claims for Clinical Chemical Methods Experiment.* NCCLS, Villanova, PA 19085, USA.

NCCLS (1984a) *Approved Guideline GP2-A: Clinical Laboratory Procedure Manuals.* NCCLS, Villanova, PA 19085, USA.

NCCLS (1984b) *Approved Guideline lG-A: Service of Clinical Laboratory Instruments.* NCCLS, Villanova, PA 19085, USA.

NCCLS (1984c) *Tentative Guideline EP5-T: User Evaluation of Precision Performance of Clinical Chemistry Devices.* NCCLS, Villanova, PA 19085, USA.

NCCLS (1984d) *Tentative Standard H18-T: Procedures for the Handling and Processing of Blood Specimens.* NCCLS, Villanova, PA 19085, USA.

Nelson, M.G. (1972) Cell counting instrument: A comparative study. In Isak, G. and Lewis, S.M. (eds.) *Modern Concepts in Hematology*, p. 201. Academic Press, New York.

Reardon, D.M., Hutchinson, D., Preston, F.E. and Trowbridge, E.A. (1985) The routine measurement of platelet volume: a comparison of aperture–impedance and flow cytometric systems. *Clin. Lab. Haematol.* **7**: 251–7.

Rowan, R.M. and Fraser, C. (1982) Platelet size distribution analysis. In van Assendelft, O.W. and England, J.M. (eds) *Advances in Hematological Methods: the Blood Count*, pp. 125–41. CRC Press, Boca Raton.

Rumke, C.L. (1978) The statistically expected variability in differential leukocyte counting. In Koepke, J.A. (ed.) *Differential Leukocyte Counting*. College of American Pathologists, Skokie, Il.

Sanders, C. and Skerry, D.W. (1961) The distribution of blood cells on haemocytometer counting chambers with special reference to the amended British Standard Specification 748. *J. Clin. Pathol.* **14**: 298.

Ward, P.J., Wardle, F. and Lewis, S.M. (1982) Standardization for routine blood counting – the role of interlaboratory trials. In Cavill, I. (ed.) *Methods in Hematology: Quality Control*, pp. 102–21. Churchill-Livingstone, Edinburgh and London.

Winkel, P., Statland, B.E., Saunders, A.M., Osborn, H. and Kupperman, H. (1981) Within-day physiologic variation of leukocyte types in healthy subjects as assayed by two automated leukocyte differential analyzers. *Am. J. Clin. Pathol.*, **75**: 693.

Chapter 5

Assessing Performance

INTRODUCTION

In the previous chapters, we have developed a description of modern hematology analyzers in terms of the technology. We have studied the history of cell counting (Chapter 1), the fundamentals of the technology (Chapter 2), described the systems (Chapter 3) and summarized the status of the development with regard to standardizing the measurements (Chapter 4). We are now ready to discuss the performance of these analytical systems. In this discussion there are two considerations. First, is the analytic performance, i.e., how well do the systems actually measure the parameters (cell count, cell size, etc.). The second is system utility, i.e., how well do the instruments perform with regard to the objective of automating the hematology laboratory.

In this chapter we will focus on the first of these considerations and discuss the analytic performance of modern cell counters relative to clinical needs and to the analytic performance of the non-automated methods that they replace. In the next chapter we will deal with the problem of integrating the system into the laboratory, combining the considerations of analytic performance of the cell counters (and their limitations) with the considerations of laboratory workflow (and its constraints).

DEFINING AN IDEAL SYSTEM

In order to develop an objective assessment of the analytic performance of modern multiparameter cell counters, either as a class (state of the art), or as individual systems, it is useful to introduce a measurable construct of an ideal system. Thus, for the purpose of assessing analytic performance, an ideal device will be defined as:

Practical Guide to Modern Hematology Analyzers. W. Groner and E. Simson
© 1995 John Wiley & Sons Ltd

A multiparameter hematology analyzer which is capable of processing all the specimens and producing results (CBC plus WBC differential) with sufficient accuracy to serve clinical needs without requiring either follow-up testing or interpretation of the results.

Unfortunately, since the modern cell counters we have described do not classify and count abnormal cells there are no modern multiparameter hematology analyzers which meet the criteria for an ideal device. Thus, in both the evaluation and integration of these instruments in the hematology laboratory one must also consider the fact that a significant number of the samples will require follow-up testing. The follow-up testing may include repeated testing after dilution and/or testing by alternative means such as visual microscopy. As a result, an important category for the performance evaluation of multiparameter cell counters must be added to account for the efficiency of the system in flagging specimens for further study.

The measurement scale for determining how close the modern systems are to the ideal can be formed by introducing two separate concepts:

1. Analytic performance.
2. Clinical sensitivity.

These concepts may in turn be defined in terms which provide the means for a practical assessment of the usefulness of modern cell counting systems:

1. *Analytic performance*. Analytic performance is measured by comparing the total analytical variation (bias plus imprecision) inherent in the results obtained from the measurement device (or system) to the biological variation which is considered clinically significant. If the analytic variation is much smaller than the biological variation it can be neglected and the results used without further consideration or testing. However, as the analytical variation approaches the biologic variation more specimens will require repeat or follow-up measurements to confirm results; thus, lowering the usefulness of the system.

2. *Clinical sensitivity*. The clinical sensitivity is the efficacy of the multi-parameter system in flagging samples for follow-up testing. Obviously, false flags will undermine the usefulness of the device. False positive flags lead to unnecessary laboratory costs while false negative flags can lead to misdiagnosis and patient mismanagement. Clinical sensitivity is measured by assessing the sensitivity and the specificity of the instrument to flag samples requiring further testing.

In the remainder of this chapter the performance of modern multi-parameter cell counters will be analyzed with regard to each of the categories defined above. In each case we will first consider the protocols by which performance is tested, then discuss the performance of individual systems, and the limitations of the state of the art. The data presented is assembled from the manufacturers, from the peer reviewed literature, and from a side by side performance evaluation conducted at our laboratory in the Long Island Jewish Medical Center on four of the most widely used multiparameter cell counting systems.

ASSESSING ANALYTIC ACCURACY

In order to evaluate system performance for analytical accuracy as defined above, it is useful to establish a meaningful quantitative scale which will separate better from good enough. Very frequently, in the absence of such a scale, relative performance claims are established by manufacturers who advertise the competitive features of their device, whether or not they are meaningful in clinical practice. This in turn can focus an evaluation on incremental improvement in the precision of a parameter (such as hemoglobin), which is already measured sufficiently precisely while other important parameters (such as the band count), which no one measures well enough, are ignored.

One valuable approach to creating such a scale for a clinical diagnostic measurement is to compare the analytical variation to biological variation. However, in applying this approach there have been some differences in exactly how to set the criteria. Various criteria defining acceptable analytic error in terms of biologic variation have been proposed by several authors over the last three decades, mainly for chemical analytes. Tonks (1963) proposed that analytic error be expressed in relation to interindividual biologic variation in health. He suggested empirically that the allowable analytical error be no more than one-fourth of the reference range for the analyte, with the reference range being expressed conventionally as twice the coefficient of variation (CV%) on either side of the mean value of a normal population, i.e. "Tonks' rule" is that the allowable analytic error is less than or equal to one-half the CV of the *interindividual* biologic variation in health (CV_i).

Cotlove (Cotlove *et al.*, 1970) proposed that desirable imprecision be less than or equal to one-half the average *within-subject* biologic variation in health. The College of American Pathologists 1976 Aspen Conference (Elevitch, 1976) recommended that the day-to-day analytical CV of a test should be less than or equal to $1/2$ CV_i for individual single and multipoint testing; they stated that this adds 11.8% or less to total observed variability. Harris (1979) provided a firm statistical footing for this goal. For group screening the CAP Aspen Conference felt that the analytical goal for imprecision (expressed as a CV) should be equal to or less than half the within-subject plus between-subject variation, which is essentially the CV of the reference range as usually obtained. Fraser in (1987) proposed that the current clinical chemistry consensus view regarding the setting of analytical goals for imprecision be adopted for hematology tests. He stated that as the goal for inaccuracy is to have no bias, analytical goals for imprecision should be used as goals for total analytic error.

In assessing the clinical accuracy of modern hematology analyzers we have taken the same general concept one step further (Simson and Groner, 1995a) by developing a more refined scale for biological variation. In this approach, rather than impose a single criterion, a set of classes is developed to grade analytic performance. We introduce a total of three categories for biological variation by considering the intraindividual biological variation in health (which is typically less than the normal or reference range), the reference range, and the total range of biologic variability encountered in patient specimens received by the laboratory (which is typically much larger than the reference or normal range). Clearly, when the total analytical variability of a measurement is small enough not to influence significantly the observed intraindividual variations (diurnal, etc.), there is no value in further improvement. The results of the measurement can be used confidently to evaluate the parameters of interest under all circumstances. At the other extreme a measurement with analytic variability comparable to the total range encountered in the laboratory will have very limited clinical value.

We can then compare the analytic variation to each level of biologic variation and create a four level measurement scale for performance of modern cell counters.

The four levels are:

Level 1

"*Ideal*". The ideal case provides maximal clinical information, as described in NCCLS H26-P (NCCLS, 1989), where the analytical CV is less than one-fourth the intraindividual biologic CV in health. This level of analytic variability contributes less than 3% to the total observed variability.

Level 2

Individual monitoring. In this case, the results are useful for evaluating a diagnosis and monitoring therapy in the individual patient, as stated at the CAP Aspen Conference (see above). This is also based on the intraindividual CV, but here the goal is that analytical CV be less than one-half the intraindividual CV. This level of analytic variability adds less than 12% to total observed variability.

Level 3

Useful for case finding (screening for disease in a population). In this case, the analytical variation is less than one-half the reference range, i.e. the interindividual CV, as defined at the Aspen Conference.

Level 4

Not useful for either individual monitoring or case finding. In this case, the analytical variability is greater than one-half the reference interval and approaches the range of variation of the analyte encountered in all the patient specimens typically tested in the laboratory.

In assessing analytic accuracy there are three independent sources of analytical variation which must be considered:

1. *System imprecision.* The fluctuations in repeated results on the same sample with the same instrument without changing the calibration.
2. *Calibration bias.* Variation of results on the same sample between systems using the same method due to the imprecision or inaccuracy of calibration.
3. *Method variation.* Variation of results obtained with different systems on the same sample due to differences in the method of analysis

In order to quantify the analytic accuracy one can study either the state of the art or the performance of a particular system. The difference between these assessments is determined by which of the three sources of analytical variation described above are included. For determining the state of the art one must include all three sources of variation. However, in assessing a particular system or class of cell counters the method variation is not included and sometimes the calibration variation is also ignored. In the following sections we shall review the analytic accuracy of multiparameter cell counters. First, we shall review the protocols which have been developed to determine analytical performance. Then, we shall review the results which have been reported in the peer reviewed literature regarding system performance. Finally, we will attempt to evaluate the state of the art, by reviewing data from interlaboratory trials and the results of a side-by-side system comparison performed at Long Island Jewish Medical Center.

PROTOCOLS FOR EVALUATING SYSTEM PERFORMANCE

Performing an evaluation for some of the key factors of analytic performance for multiparameter cell counters is within the capability of the individual laboratory. Protocols have been established which aid in the collection of data and the comparison of results. Of particular interest is the evaluation of *precision* (to determine the within run and day-to-day variation of an individual cell counter) and the evaluation of *comparability* (to determine the comparison between the results of a cell counter system and the system in current routine use). The protocols which are described briefly below follow the recommendations of the ICSH expert panel on cytometry in "Guidelines for the evaluation of blood cell analyzers including those used for differential leukocyte and reticulocyte counting and cell marker applications" (ICSH, 1984; ICSH, 1994) and those of NCCLS (NCCLS, 1982a,b,c, 1984d).

Evaluating precision

Precision is established by testing a sample on two or more occasions. Precision may be quantified using the standard deviation of the repeated results or the coefficient of variation defined as the standard deviation divided by the mean. It is usual to consider precision when the sample is assayed repeatedly within one batch of samples (within-batch or replicate precision), as well as when the sample is assayed in separate batches (between batch, or day-to-day precision). However, since blood specimens are less stable in general than cell counters, it is impractical to study anything other than replicate precision of automated blood cell counters with fresh whole blood samples. As a result, practical evaluation of the precision of multiparameter cell counters generally involves two separate studies: one in which fresh whole blood samples are replicated within the batch, preferably not immediately after each other, and one in which the day-to-day variability of the cell counter is assayed using stabilized surrogate blood materials.

Ideally, precision studies should be performed over the whole pathological range. Separate batches of specimens should certainly be analyzed in duplicate representing the high, low and normal range of each parameter. Similarly, in assessing day-to-day precision, stabilized test material representing high, medium and low values should be analyzed daily for a period not less than thirty days. Analysis of paired results is done by dividing the standard deviation of the difference between pairs by the batch mean while analysis of repeated results on a single specimen is performed by dividing the standard deviation by the mean.

It should be noted that these two methods of analysis are not equivalent. In one case the difference is between pairs while in the other it is the difference from the mean. Thus, due only to the definition of the analysis, the data from paired results for short-term imprecision will be 1.4 times greater than that obtained by replicated sampling of a single specimen.

Evaluating comparability between instruments

Comparability may be defined generally as the ability of the instrument under test to produce results which agree satisfactorily with those obtained by routine current procedures; or with a reference method. Typically, modern hematology analyzers may need to have one or more parameters calibrated with suitable material. Instrument evaluation can be badly affected by this limitation since it can be difficult to decide whether a blood counter is working incorrectly or has been calibrated with a material whose assigned values are incorrect. For example: if counter A always gave values 10% greater than counter B this could be quite acceptable if the difference is easily eliminated by correct calibration. It would be unacceptable, however, if counter A gave answers 5% higher on some samples and 50% higher on others: in this instance there would be a serious variation only 5% of which could be attributed to calibration.

The ICSH guidelines (see above) for the evaluation of comparability between instruments are paraphrased below:

- In evaluating comparability as many routine samples should be studied as possible; the results should be analyzed by a paired t-test and presented as a graph of the difference between methods plotted as a function of the level of the parameter under test. Table 5.1 shows an example for a small number of observations of the packed cell volume (PCV).
- If the unselected series of routine samples does not give sufficient information about samples at the extremes of the pathological range such samples should be selected and studied in detail separately. The full range expected in clinical practice must be studied. However, the result obtained with selected samples should not be merged when performing the statistical analysis with those in the unselected series since this would bias the statistical sampling. The results from special samples, however, may be included in the graphical representation.
- When the comparability study exposes discrepant results, the samples should be studied by reference methods to identify the cause. If reference methods are not available attempts should still be made to resolve discrepancies by using methods which the evaluator considers will be sufficiently accurate and precise.

Table 5.1 Calculation of comparability between test and reference methods: a numerical example for PCV (n = 5) expressed as a fraction

Sample no.	Result current method	Result test method	Difference (*d*)
1	0.281	0.249	0.032
2	0.422	0.361	0.061
3	0.489	0.383	0.106
4	0.417	0.345	0.072
5	0.472	0.393	0.079

$\Sigma\, d$ = 0.35
$\Sigma\, d^2$ = 0.0276
$\Sigma\, d/n$ = 0.07.

- Comparisons between the method under test and the method in current use should also be made with material obtained from a national external quality assessment scheme or interlaboratory trials. The results will give an indication of the test instrument's performance as compared with others and also the ability of the instrument to use materials which are supplied in the interlaboratory surveys.
- Table 5.2 lists some of the important potential interferences for hematology analyzers. In the comparability studies as many unselected samples as possible are tested in order to represent the full range expected in clinical practice. However, the relatively rare samples with the abnormalities listed in the table which are known to be a potential interference may not have been included. If this is so, a special study should be made of the instrument's response to such abnormal samples and interference.
- In addition to the abnormal samples and interference studies the protocol should also test known measurement interferences such as the effect of microcytosis on platelet counts, and of leukocytosis on the hemoglobin determination. If possible these should be studied separately in dose response experiments performed with manipulated samples.

Evaluating comparability to the microscope

Typically, when an automated multiparameter cell counter capable of producing a full five part WBC differential is first introduced into the laboratory the method in routine use for the WBC differential is the visual evaluation of the peripheral blood film. This method is generally limited by the number of cells counted and therefore the imprecision of the routine method may be substantially greater than the instrument

Table 5.2 Abnormal samples and interferents requiring study

Abnormal samples	Interferents
Hemoglobin S and C	Hemolysis in vitro
Nucleated red blood cells	Micro-clots
Heinz and Howell Jolly bodies	Cold agglutinins
Malarial parasites	Paraproteinemia
Red cell fragments	Hyperbilirubinemia
Atypical lymphocytes	Lipemia
Immature white blood cells	Uremia
Giant platelets	Non-ketotic hyperosmolarity

From ICSH (1984) with permission.

under test. Further, although the automated instrument may also present the results of the differential count in terms of the number of cells per unit volume the microscopic method can only report the results as a fraction of the total population.

The NCCLS has considered this problem and issued a document (H20-A) which defines the reference differential for visual microscopy and gives guidelines for analyzing the data when an automated instrument is compared to a microscope differential (NCCLS, 1992). In analyzing the data from such an experiment, the simple paired t-test described above for use with the traditional CBC parameters is insufficient and one must consider whether the differences in counts can be explained by the combined imprecision of the test and reference methods or whether they represent true differences between the methods. To perform this analysis a statistical model is built which predicts the standard error between the test method and the routine method that is expected solely as a result of the imprecision of the methods. The statistical analysis of this situation has been made (Rumke, 1978) and Figure 5.1 shows graphically the expected standard error as a function of the percentage of cells (SEp). Curves which represent the 95% confidence limits between the cell counter results and visual microscopy are shown for several representative numbers of cell classified by microscopy. The NCCLS recommends that for the purpose of evaluating the comparability of automated cell counters the reference method should be a 400 cell visual differential. This represents a compromise between the imprecision of lower numbers of cells and the impracticality of higher numbers. However, at this level the imprecision of the reference method is still greater than that of the system under test and this may limit the evaluation. As an example, Figures 5.2 to 5.6 show the results obtained when each of four multiparameter systems were compared to a 400 cell microscope differential on a series of approximately 500 samples. In each case the confidence interval (95%) based on the counting statistics is superimposed on

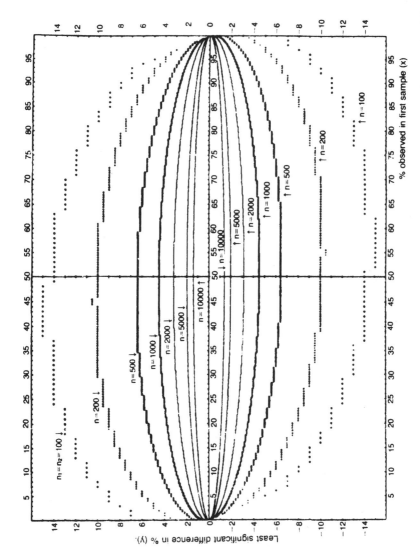

Figure 5.1 Expected standard errors as a function of the percentage of cells (SEp). From Rumke (1978) with permission

the data. It is seen in analyzing these data that each of the instruments compares fairly well for each of the cell types. Table 5.3 summarizes the regression parameters for the comparability between the four analyzers and the 400 cell microscopic reference differential. The last column in the table gives the percentage of points which fall within the confidence interval defined by the imprecision of sampling. It can be seen that for each analyzer and each cell type, approximately 95% of the results fall within the confidence interval. Thus, the results from each of the analyzers are comparable to the microscopic differential.

SYSTEM ANALYTIC PERFORMANCE RESULTS

Results regarding the analytic performance of modern cell counter systems are available from either of two independent sources. Instrument evaluations performed by individual laboratories (or regional assessment groups) are reported in the peer reviewed literature, and the results of interlaboratory trials are summarized periodically. In the following paragraphs we shall briefly review the reported results.

Instrument evaluations

Evaluations of modern instruments have been reported in many journal articles generally following the protocols which were described above. Most of these evaluations focus on the imprecision of the instruments and the relation between one particular instrument's performance and the microscope results for the WBC differential in that laboratory. Since the laboratory specimens and the methods of reporting results are generally specific to each study it is sometimes difficult to compare results and an impression of wide variation in performance is given, especially with regard to the automated WBC differential. However, recently reports of comparisons between pairs or groups of systems have also been issued. These reports show much less variation between the results obtained with different systems than would be implied from the individual instrument evaluation reports.

Table 5.4 summarizes results reported in 14 separate evaluations of the within-run imprecision of modern cell counting systems with regard to the eight standard CBC parameters. It can be seen from the table that the reported imprecision for these parameters is uniform with an average CV of 1% or less for the red blood cell parameters, approximately 2% for the WBC count and 2.3% for the platelet count.

Table 5.5 summarizes the results reported in 15 separate evaluations of one or more modern cell counters with regard to the within-run imprecision of the five components of the WBC differential. The data contained in Table 5.5 shows somewhat greater variation than noted in

a   **H*1 vs. Manual Reference Neutrophil Count**

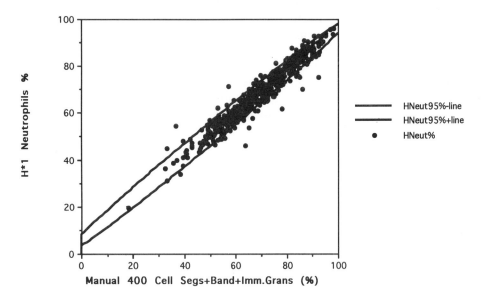

b   **CellDyn 3000 vs. Manual Reference Neutrophil Count**

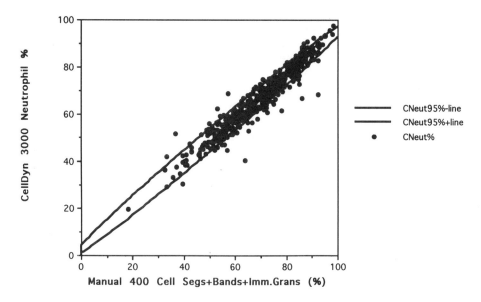

Figure 5.2 Comparison of automated differential analyzers for neutrophils. Each analyzer is compared to the 400 cell reference differential. Regression parameters are listed in Table 5.3. a) H*1, b) CellDyn 3000, c) NE8000, d) STKS

c   **NE8000 vs. Manual Reference Neutrophil Count**

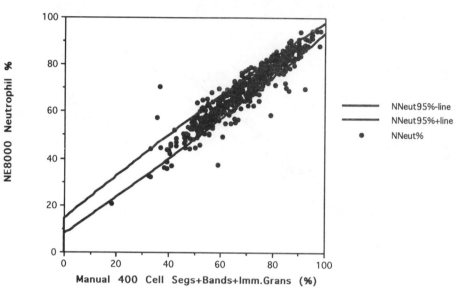

d   **STKS vs. Manual Reference Neutrophil Count**

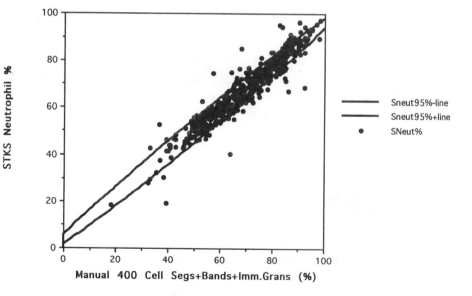

a CellDyn 3000 vs. Manual Reference Lymphocyte Count

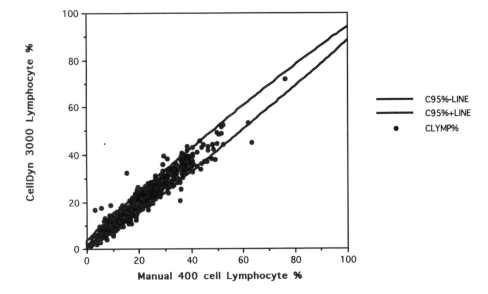

b   H*1 vs. Manual Reference Lymphocyte Count

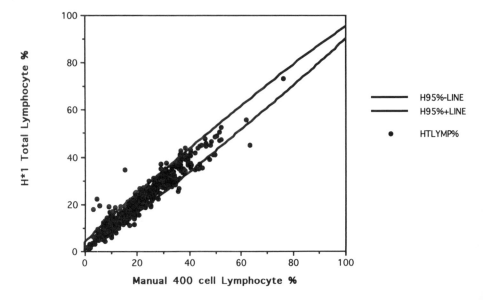

Figure 5.3 Comparison of automated differential analyzers for lymphocytes. Each analyzer is compared to the 400 cell reference differential. Regression parameters are listed in Table 5.3. a) CellDyn 3000, b) H*1, c) STKS, d) NE8000

c   **STKS vs. Manual Reference Lymphocyte Count**

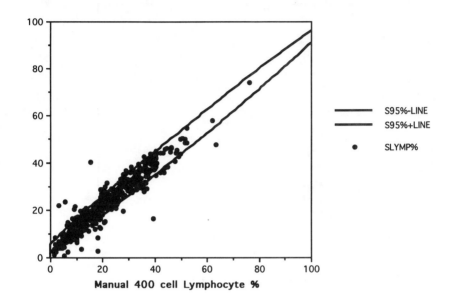

d   **NE8000 vs. Manual Reference Lymphocyte Count**

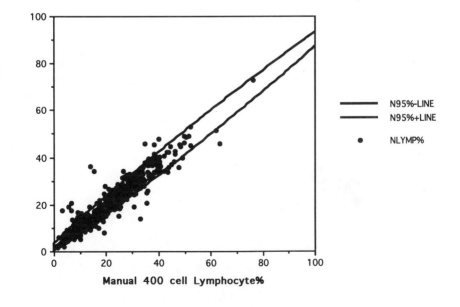

a   CellDyn 3000 vs. Manual Reference Monocyte Count

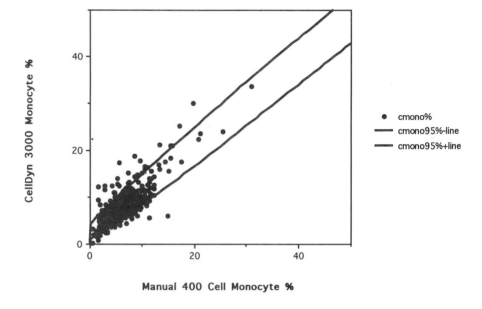

b   H*1 vs. Manual Reference Monocyte Count

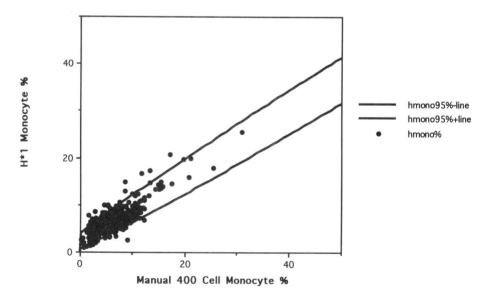

Figure 5.4   Comparison of automated differential analyzers for monocytes. Each analyzer is compared to the 400 cell reference differential. Regression parameters are listed in Table 5.3. a) CellDyn 3000, b) H*1, c) STKS, d) NE8000

c **STKS vs. Manual Reference Monocyte Count**

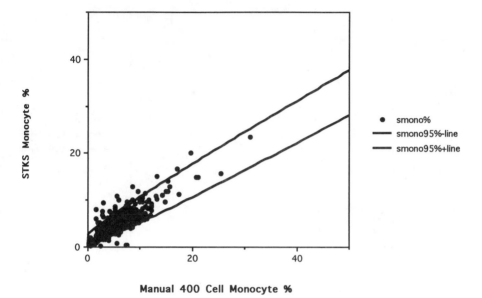

d **NE8000 vs. Manual Reference Monocyte Count**

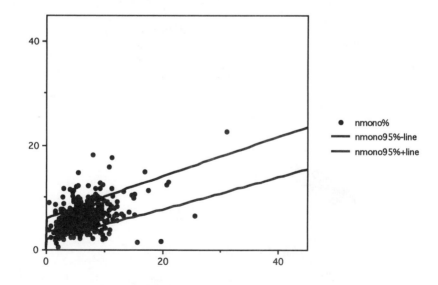

a   **CellDyn 3000 vs. Manual Reference Eosinophil Count**

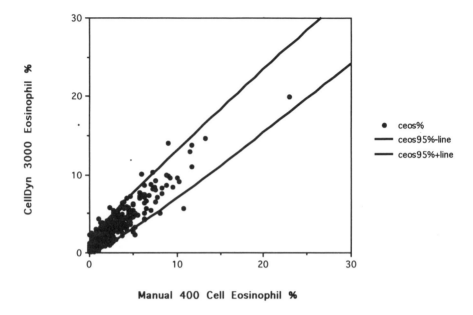

b   **H*1 vs. Manual Reference Eosinophil Count**

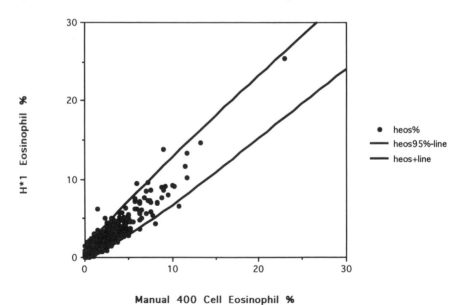

Figure 5.5 Comparison of automated differential analyzers for eosinophils. Each analyzer is compared to the 400 cell reference differential. Regression parameters are listed in Table 5.3. a) CellDyn 3000, b) H*1, c) NE8000, d) STKS

c   **NE8000 vs. Manual Reference Eosinophil Count**

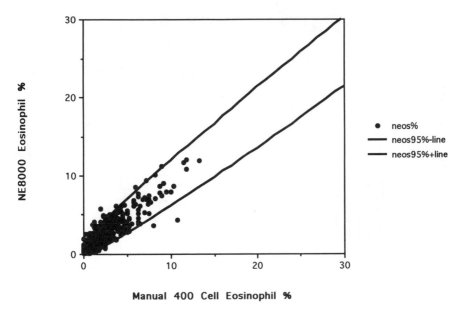

d   **STKS vs. Manual Reference Eosinophil Count**

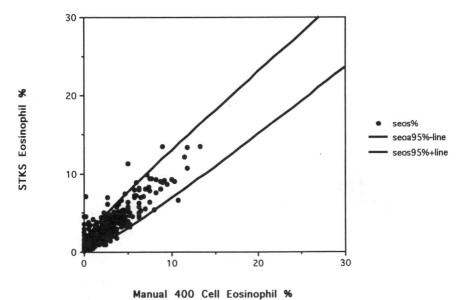

a   CellDyn 3000 vs. Manual Reference Basophil Count

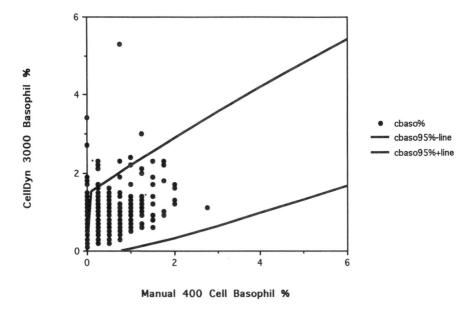

b   H*1 Basophils vs. Manual Reference Basophil Count

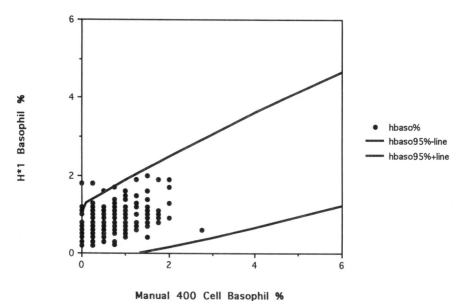

Figure 5.6 Comparison of automated differential analyzers for basophils. Each analyzer is compared to the 400 cell reference differential. Regression parameters are listed in Table 5.3. a) CellDyn 3000, b) H*1, c) NE8000, d) STKS

c   **NE8000 vs. Manual Reference Basophil Count**

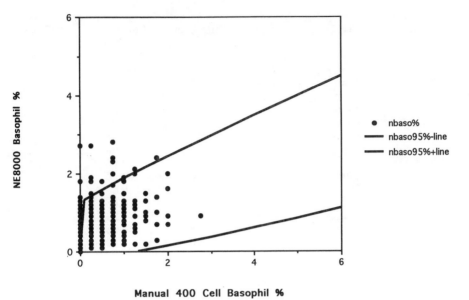

Manual 400 Cell Basophil %

d   **STKS vs. Manual Reference Basophil Count**

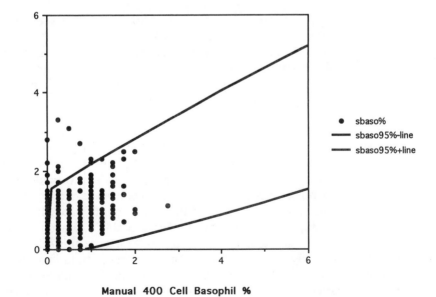

Manual 400 Cell Basophil %

Table 5.3 Summary of regression parameters for four analyzers vs 400 cell reference

System	Cell type	Slope	Intercept	Correlation coefficient r^2	% Within sample error
STKS	Neut	0.92	3.5	0.91	94.4
H*1	Neut	0.90	5.9	0.93	96.8
NE-8000	Neut	0.84	11.0	0.88	92.7
CD-3000	Neut	0.92	2.7	0.93	96.0
STKS	Lymph	0.90	3.66	0.95	92.9
H*1	Lymph*	0.90	2.31	0.96	95.2
NE-8000	Lymph	0.88	1.94	0.95	92.9
CD-3000	Lymph	0.89	1.90	0.96	94.7
STKS	Mono	0.62	1.5	0.65	95.9
H*1	Mono	0.68	2.3	0.66	97.8
NE-8000	Mono	0.34	3.9	0.20	91.7
CD-3000	Mono	0.91	2.5	0.63	95.8
STKS	Eos	0.91	0.67	0.80	97.0
H*1	Eos	0.94	0.20	0.87	97.6
NE-8000	Eos	0.84	0.56	0.81	98.3
CD-3000	Eos	0.94	0.60	0.85	98.7
STKS	Baso	0.48	0.53	0.19	98.4
H*1	Baso	0.41	0.49	0.31	99.6
NE-8000	Baso	0.37	0.52	0.13	97.8
CD-3000	Baso	0.49	0.62	0.18	97.8

*Includes large unstained cells (LUC).

Table 5.4. However, there is no significant difference between instruments when a Student t-test is applied to the reported results between the instruments of different manufacturers, and those reports in which more than one instrument was compared showed less variation in imprecision. Thus, whatever differences exist cannot be obtained from the literature, especially from manufacturer claims or single instrument evaluations.

In Table 5.5 the imprecision is also compared to the imprecision of a reference visual differential of 200 cells. It is seen that in general, the imprecision of the automated differential counters is approximately one-third that of a manual 200 cell differential. This is roughly consistent with the increase in the number of cells counted (typically between 2000 and 10 000) by the automated differential counter. Recall that the imprecision of sampling is given by the reciprocal of the square root of the number of cells counted. Thus, an improvement in imprecision by a factor of 3 is roughly equivalent to an order of magnitude increase (i.e. × 10) in the number of cells classified. Monocytes in Table 5.5 are the only cell to demonstrate improvement of less than a factor of three.

Table 5.4 Within-run imprecision of eight hematology parameters (summary of reported results*)

Parameter	Lowest value CV %	Highest value CV %	Average value CV %
Hemoglobin	0.4	0.8	0.55
RBC count	0.4	1.1	0.65
PCV	0.4	1.3	0.78
MCV	0.2	1.2	0.51
MCH	0.4	3.8	1.0
MCHC	0.6	1.5	0.95
Platelet count	1.1	3.9	2.31
WBC count	1.4	3.4	1.90

*Summary of 14 reported results.
  Coulter = 5
  Sysmex = 4
  Abbott = 3
  Bayer = 2
Difference between manufacturers not significant.

Table 5.5 Within-run imprecision of the automated leukocyte differential (summary of reported data*)

Cell type	Lowest value	Highest value	Average value	Manual[†] (200 cell)	Ratio man/avge
Neut (CV %)	0.7	4.17	1.74	5.6	3.21
Lymph (CV %)	1.1	4.08	2.50	8.6	3.44
Mono (CV %)	4.0	63.3	13.5	25.9	1.91
Eos (CV %)	6.3	43.8	12.9	39.3	3.0
Baso (CV %)	6.6	76.6	31.8	96.3	3.0

*From 15 reports
  4 = Coulter method
  4 = TOA method
  3 = Bayer method
  3 = Abbott method
  1 = Roche method
Differences between manufacturers not significant.
[†]Data from Buttarello *et al.* (1992).

This implies that other sources of imprecision in monocyte counting are substantive and greater than the imprecision of sampling.

Table 5.6 summarizes the reported results of 15 regression experiments between the microscope and automated differential counters. Here again, it is impossible with a Student *t*-test to distinguish between systems of one manufacturer and another on the basis of the data. It is also noted that correlation for monocytes and basophils is

Table 5.6 Summary of reported correlation data* on accuracy of the automated leukocyte differential

Cell type	Lowest value (coeff, r)	Highest value (coeff, r)	Average value (coeff, r)
Neut	0.88	0.99	0.96
Lymph	0.89	0.99	0.95
Mono	0.26	0.89	0.60
Eos	0.69	0.98	0.90
Baso	0.00	0.60	0.35

*From 15 reports
  4 = Coulter method
  4 = TOA method
  3 = Bayer method
  3 = Abbott method
  1 = Roche method
Differences between methods not significant.

generally poor. Poor correlation for these cell types was also observed in the studies which were used as an example in the previous section on measuring comparability to the microscope. However, it cannot be determined whether this is a result of sampling error, poor visual recognition and/or a limitation on the performance of automated counters since approximately 95% of the results fell within the confidence interval for sampling error.

Interlaboratory trials

The analytical variability for a particular system or group of systems from the same manufacturer, as reported in the literature does not include the third component (method see p. 123) of among-system variation and therefore does not allow an assessment of the state of the art. To assess the total variation and determine the state of the art one must resort to the data from either interlaboratory trials or multiple system side-by-side evaluations. Interlaboratory trials are conducted periodically by several organizations, including manufacturers, national organizations such as UKNEQAS (United Kingdom National External Quality Assessment Scheme), and professional organizations such as CAP (College of American Pathologists). These results are summarized periodically in the literature. In general these trials are conducted using stabilized blood specimens and as indicated in the previous chapter matrix effects associated with those materials still limit the interpetation of results. Consequently, only results with regard to the traditional CBC are useful in comparing systems. Table 5.7 summarizes the results of 10 consecutive NEQAS trials for the eight parameter CBC and com-

Table 5.7 Typical interlaboratory trial results (SI units) for hematology parameters

Parameter	Trial specimen range of values*	Total CV % range*	Total CV % average*	Total CV % over precision	Average imprecision CV %[†]
Hemoglobin	113.0–125.0	1.22–1.91	1.49	2.7	0.55
Red cell count	3.80–4.57	1.46–1.76	1.60	2.46	0.65
PCV	0.345–0.427	2.78–3.62	3.31	4.24	0.78
MCV	89.1–93.1	2.01–2.45	2.23	4.37	0.51
MCH	29.2–30.2	1.76–2.24	1.97	1.97	1.0
MCHC	32.4–34.9	3.15–3.58	3.38	3.55	0.95
White cell count	5.5–8.3	5.36–8.79	6.64	2.87	2.31
Platelet count	172–271	5.24–9.81	6.55	3.44	1.90

*Taken over 10 sequential NEQAS trials (1992–1993).
[†]Taken from Table 5.4.

pares the total CV to the average within-run CV reported in Table 5.4. The limited geographic area of the United Kingdom and the rapid delivery methods employed allow UKNEQAS to use material with relatively small matrix effects. In Table 5.7 averages have been taken over all of the automated systems for each of the eight parameters. As in the results reported above on individual instrument evaluations, there is no statistically significant difference between the results of any particular manufacturer or system. Further, it is seen that the total variation is generally three times larger than the within-run imprecision. Thus, the components of calibrator bias and method variation are larger contributors to the total variation than the within-run imprecision.

Results for the components of the WBC differential from some interlaboratory trials performed on several of the major modern systems have now also become available to participants. These trials are performed with stabilized materials that are designed to be compatible with the systems under test. Thus, different materials are used for different manufacturer's systems and results can only be compared for one type of system. Further, the stabilized materials are still undergoing revision and consequently results are not yet consistent enough to use in reviewing performance of the modern cell counters with regard to the WBC differential.

STATE OF THE ART FOR ANALYTIC ACCURACY

In order to determine the state of the art for a measurement parameter one needs to assess the total variation that could be expected on the results of a series of typical blood samples due to all three sources of analytic variation listed above (imprecision, calibration bias and method variation) and compare that to the biological variation. This is conceptually easy but it is usually very difficult to conduct a good experiment on modern cell counters for two related reasons. The first reason is the lability of the specimen which precludes obtaining many results on the same specimen. The second reason is the scarcity of data on the biological variability of hematology parameters (most probably due to the problems in specimen handling).

Much work has been done on the generation and application of data on biological variation in clinical chemistry analytes; estimates of intraindividual and between-person variation now exist for more than 150 chemistry analytes (Fraser and Petersen, 1993). However, there are much less data for the hematology parameters. There are comprehensive data on interindividual variation (reference ranges) for various ages for both CBC and WBC differential parameters in nationwide studies in the United States and worldwide in the book by Bain (1989), which has a compilation of data from 85 publications. However, very few data on intraindividual biologic variation for hematologic analytes appear in the literature.

Studies on long-term (9 months and one year) biological variability on CBC measurements (Ross *et al.*, 1988; Dot *et al.*, 1992) and a study of CBC and three part differential values in the elderly (Fraser *et al.*, 1989) have been published. For short-term (within-day and day-to-day variation), there are two separate studies by Statland and Winkel (Statland, 1977; Winkel, 1981), one on 20, the other on 21 normal subjects, and an as yet unpublished study by Richardson-Jones *et al.* on 34 subjects (Richardson-Jones, personal communication 1994).

The averages of the reported values for biologic variability of the hematology parameters are summarized in Table 5.8. It is seen in Table 5.8 that the intraindividual biological variation is roughly associated with the length of time the cells spend in the circulation. The six red blood cell parameters have the least biologic variability, which may be related to the 90–120 day life span of the RBC. Thus, the intraindividual variations for these parameters are 3% or less. The much shorter lived platelet (–10 days) has an intraindividual variation of 6% while the even shorter lived WBCs (e.g. 8 hours for granulocytes) have even larger intraindividual variations.

Typically, the ratio of approximately 3 obtains between the intraindividual and interindividual variations of hematology parameters. Note that the typical laboratory range is another factor of two bringing the total range between laboratory variability and intraindividual variability to between six and ten. Thus, the dimensions of the scale which has been defined to estimate the state of the art have approximately one

Table 5.8 Biological variation of hematology parameters

Parameter	Intraindividual range CV %**	Interindividual range CV %*	Laboratory range CV %†
Hemoglobin	2.5	8.4	18.6
RBC	3.2	9.0	19.2
PCV	2.1	6.9	20.2
MCV	1.0	4.8	9.2
MCH	0.4	4.9	9.1
MCHC	0.6	2.9	2.3
WBC	13.0	22.3	62.9
Platelet	6.0	20.9	44.9
RDW	1.0	5.4	16.8
Neut (%)	5.6	12.8	19.3
Lymph (%)	8.9	21.2	53.1
Mono (%)	9.3	24.3	37.5
Eos (%)	25.6	63.1	93.7
Baso (%)	17.9	42.2	50.4
Neut (Abs)	14.8	30.8	69.3
Lymph (Abs)	11.6	31.1	56.0
Mono (Abs)	15.3	29.5	54.2
Eos (Abs)	22.0	70.1	104.9
Baso (Abs)	12.4	46.6	51.9
MPV		9.8	
PDW		3.6	

*From a 120 specimen normal study performed at Long Island Jewish Medical Center (LIJ).
†From a series of 545 specimens encountered in the routine laboratory at LIJ.
**From Statland, Winkel and Richardson-Jones (see text).

order of magnitude in total variability between ideal performance and essentially useless numbers.

The eight parameter CBC

The most common means of estimating the total analytic variation among systems is through interlaboratory trials, as discussed above. In these studies a small number of artificially preserved samples are transported and analyzed on a large number of different systems, the results are then compared and the variability is calculated.

As a first example, consider the measurement of hemoglobin: Tables 5.7 and 5.9 show typical results of interlaboratory trials for hemoglobin performed in the UK by the UKNEQAS. These show a total analytic variation, including among system variation, of 1.5–1.6%. The interindividual variation in hemoglobin is about 9% (Table 5.8), and the intraindividual variation is about 2.5%. Thus, the state of the art for the

Table 5.9   Typical interlaboratory trial results* for hemoglobin

System group	N	Median	SD	CV %
Coulter S+ systems	265	138.0	1.48	1.07
Roche systems	32	138.0	2.59	1.89
Bayer systems	158	138.0	1.48	1.07
TOA systems	59	140.0	1.48	1.06
Semiautomated	42	139.5	2.97	2.13
All systems	922	139.0	2.22	1.60

*UKNEQAS survey 9312, partially fixed human blood.
Value by ICSH reference method 139.0.

among system determination of hemoglobin is greater than one-fourth the intraindividual variation but less than both one-fourth and one-half the interindividual variation and falls into the third class defined above (useful for case finding only). It is also noted in Table 5.9 that the total within-system variation for automated hemoglobin measurement is approximately 1% for most manufacturers. Therefore, performance for these automated systems falls into class 2 i.e. suitable for individual monitoring also. However, the variation for semiautomated methods is greater than 2%, putting them in the third category.

In summary: modern automated hematology analyzers represent the state of the art for the determination of hemoglobin, while semiautomated systems fall a little short. Automated multiparameter systems can be used both for tracking individuals and for case finding with regard to this parameter. However, ideal performance (total analytic variation less than one-fourth the intraindividual biologic variation) is not yet attainable principally due to the small biologic variation in hemoglobin.

The results of interlaboratory trials can be used in a similar manner to determine the state of the art for the other parameters of the CBC, such as hematocrit, white blood cell count, red blood cell count, mean cell volume, and the platelet count. Table 5.7 lists typical results for these parameters averaged over ten consecutive UKNEQAS trials.

The results in Tables 5.8 and 5.7 can now be used for a comparison for these eight parameters between the total analytical variation from interlaboratory trials and the biological variation. This is done in Table 5.10 where the total analytical variation is divided by the biological variation at each of three levels. It is seen that for none of these eight parameters is the analytic variation small enough to reach the ideal (class 1) where the total analytic variation is 1/4 the intraindividual variation. For four of the eight parameters (hemoglobin, RBC, WBC and platelets) the total variation is small compared to the interindivi-

Table 5.10 State of the art: analytic variation (total)/biological variation of eight hematology parameters

Parameter	Total variability CV %*	Total/intra- range†	Total/inter range†	Total/lab range†	Performance level
Hb	1.49	0.60	0.18	0.08	3
RBC	1.6	0.50	0.18	0.08	2
PCV	3.31	1.58	0.48	0.16	3
MCV	2.23	2.23	0.46	0.24	3
MCH	1.97	4.93	0.40	0.22	3
MCHC	3.38	5.63	1.17	1.47	4
WBC	6.64	0.51	0.30	0.11	2
Platelet	6.55	1.09	0.31	0.15	3

*Analytic variability from Table 5.7.
†Biological variability from Table 5.8.

dual biologic variation in health. However, for one parameter (MCHC) the total analytic variation is equivalent to the total laboratory range lending credibility to the generally held concept that laboratory findings in this parameter are meaningless (Rose, 1971).

In summary, the state of the art for these eight parameters is represented by the modern cell counters and the principal source of analytical variation is not the imprecision of counting but calibration bias and method variation. The results for RBC and WBC are useful for both case finding and tracking and the others (with the exception of MCHC) are useful for case finding. However, with the exception of the WBC the biologic variation of these parameters is so small that even the relatively small analytic variation falls short of the criteria for an ideal measurement.

The automated differential

Assessing the state of the art for the automated differential is more difficult due to sparse data on both total analytic and biologic variation. The ability to assess the total analytic variation through the results of interlaboratory trials is only useful for those parameters where a representative sample can be prepared for distribution and analysis. Unfortunately, this is not the case for WBC differential parameters reported by modern hematology analyzers. Although each system is calibrated with whole blood it is not practical to use whole blood for interlaboratory trials and the available stabilized materials show marked differences (matrix effects) when analyzed on different systems. Consequently, the total analytic variability of the components of the leukocyte differential and the cell size parameters (RDW, PDW, MPV) are not easily obtained as they are not often subjected to typical interlaboratory trials. As pointed out above, limited results of interlaboratory trials are available for the components of the WBC differential obtained with special materials tailored for use with a particular cell counting system. These trials allow an estimate of the analytic variability for a particular class of cell counters but do not allow an estimate of the state of the art.

One means of making an assessment of the total variability for these parameters is by running a series of fresh blood samples on an example of each of the major cell counting systems and comparing the results. The results are then analyzed in a manner analogous to the determination of comparability between two methods with the CV across the analyzers replacing the difference between methods. In this case a relatively large number of samples are compared on a relatively small number of systems. As this is a rather difficult experiment it has only been done a few times. The results of one such experiment which was conducted at Long Island Jewish Medical Center (LIJ) is shown in Figures 5.7 to 5.11 where the variation across four instruments is plotted against the level. In this study approximately 500 specimens were tested on each of four analyzers (Coulter STKS, TOA NE-8000, Technicon H*1, and Abbott CD-3000). The figures demonstrate the frequency distribution of the analytic variation for each of the five components of the WBC differential as reported on the cell counting systems. In order to make the results comparable for lymphocytes, the LUC count from the Technicon H*1 was added to the lymphocytes.

Results for the same set of specimens were calculated in a similar manner for the components of the eight parameter CBC. Thus for these parameters there are two means of assessing the total analytic variability, and it is interesting to compare the results obtained by the different methods.

Table 5.11 (p. 154) compares the average CV obtained in the system comparisons experiment to the CV obtained in interlaboratory trials for the parameters of the CBC. It is seen that for the parameters where both means of assessing the total analytic variability are available they give approximately the same results.

Table 5.12 determines the state of the art for the WBC differential parameters. This is done by comparing the total analytic variability obtained by taking the average value for the variance across the four cell counters for each of the five classes of leukocyte as determined in the system comparisons experiments, to the biologic variability both as percentage and absolute values. It is seen that none of the parameters reaches the ideal level, and in fact only neutrophils reach the class 2 level. It is further noted that the total analytic variability of both mono-

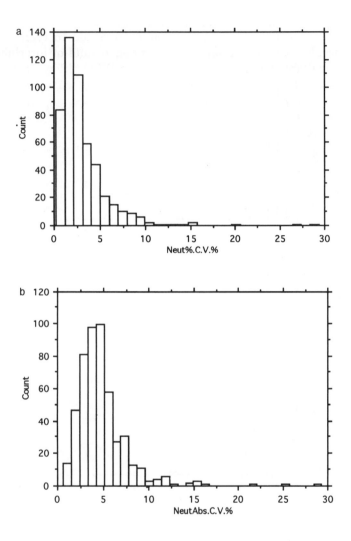

Figure 5.7 Distribution of analytical variability for (a) percentage neutrophils and (b) absolute neutrophils

cytes and basophils approaches the levels of laboratory variability therefore limiting the clinical utility of these parameters.

Table 5.13 (p. 155) compares the total variability of the five white cell classes to the average duplicate imprecision obtained in the same study. It is seen from this table that with the exception of basophils the dominant factor in the total analytic variability results from the differences in cell classification methods. Method bias is approximately three

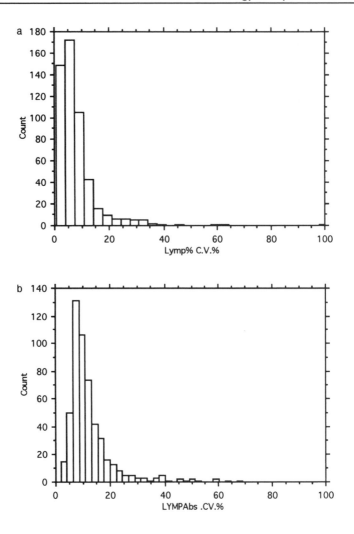

Figure 5.8 Distribution of analytical variability for (a) percentage lymphocytes and (b) absolute lymphocytes

times the imprecision. Thus, to a large degree the increases in precision
afforded by automation of the WBC differential have been offset by differences in the technology of cell classification.

In spite of these results it is still interesting to compare the total
variability as observed in the system trials to the sampling error (SEp)
of the manual differential at various cell count levels; and to compare
this with the expected sampling error of the 400 cell manual reference
differential. To perform this comparison the coefficients of variation

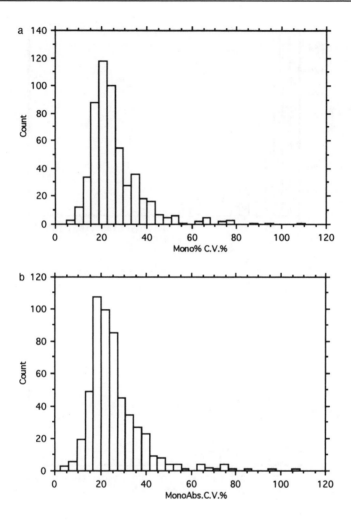

Figure 5.9 Distribution of analytical variability for (a) percentage monocytes and (b) absolute monocytes

(CV) for percentage differential counts obtained from the system variability study are shown in Figures 5.12–5.16 with curves superimposed on them illustrating the differences which would be expected from sampling error for each of the five white blood cell types. The standard error (SEp) for sampling levels of 200 cells, 400 cells, 2000 cells, and 10 000 cells are illustrated. Table 5.14 gives the percentage of results which fall within the sampling error at sampling levels of 200, 400, 600, 800, 1000, 1500, 2000 and 10 000 cells. If the observed variability

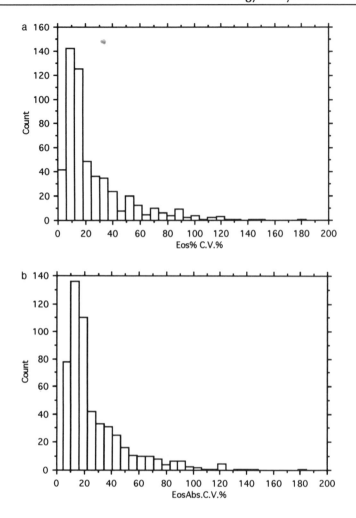

Figure 5.10 Distribution of analytical variability for (a) percentage eosinophils and (b) absolute eosinophils

at a particular level of cell count were due solely to sampling error, 95%
or more of results would fall within the limits. As the average WBC
count for the series of samples studied was 11 500 and the mode and
median approximately 8000, the 10 000 cell level is closest to the
number of cells typically classified by the analyzers for the samples in
this study. Figures 5.12–5.16 and Table 5.14 show that at the 400 cell
level, all cell types are within the sampling error level and at 600 cells,
all cell types except monocytes at 91.7% are well above the 95% limit.

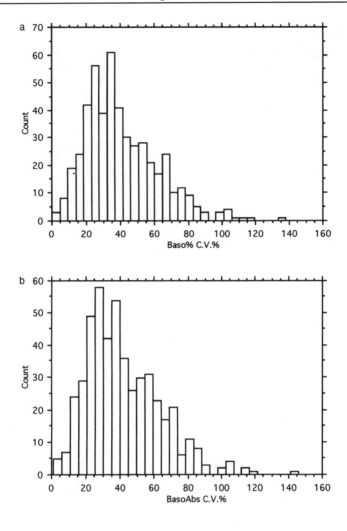

Figure 5.11 Distribution of analytical variability for (a) percentage basophils and (b) absolute basophils

All cell types except monocytes at 86.5% are within the error levels at 800 cells. At 1000 cells, neutrophils drop to 92.5% and lymphocytes to 94.1%; at 1500 cells, all cell types are below the 95% cut-off except eosinophils at 95.2%. Thus, this analysis shows that the variability among analyzers is far greater than would be expected for sampling error alone and methodologic differences probably play a role.

For all five cell types the analytic variability of the automated differential is less than would be expected for the variation solely due to

Table 5.11 Comparison of total variability data: Interlaboratory trials vs system comparisons

	Interlaboratory trials		System comparisons	
Parameter	Specimen range*	CV % average	Specimen range†	CV % average
Hemoglobin	113.0–125.0	1.49	51.8–177.3	1.23
RBC	3.80–4.57	1.60	1.64–7.54	1.51
PCV	0.345–0.427	3.31	0.15–0.637	2.27
MCV	89.1–93.1	2.23	58.7–113.4	1.71
MCH	29.2–30.2	1.97	18.8–38.98	1.95
MCHC	32.4–34.9	3.38	30.1–36.2	2.72
WBC	5.5–8.3	6.64	1.9–56.9	4.94
Platelet count	172–271	6.55	36–900	6.03

*10 NEQAS samples with between 800 and 900 systems reporting.
†650 samples with four systems reporting.

Table 5.12 State of the art: Analytic variation (total)/biological variation of automated differential parameters

Parameter	Total variability CV %	Total/intra range	Total/inter range	Total/lab range	Performance level
Neut (%)	3.14	0.56	0.25	0.16	3
Lymph (%)	10.1	1.13	0.46	0.19	3
Mono (%)	26.0	2.80	1.07	0.69	4
Eos (%)	26.3	1.03	0.42	0.28	3
Baso (%)	41.0	2.29	0.97	0.81	4
Neut (Abs)	4.96	0.34	0.16	0.07	2
Lymph (Abs)	12.4	1.07	0.40	0.25	3
Mono (Abs)	26.0	1.70	0.88	0.48	4
Eos (Abs)	28.7	1.30	0.41	0.27	3
Baso (Abs)	41.9	3.38	0.90	0.81	4

sampling in a 400 cell differential and, despite method differences, is at the 800–1000 cell level except for monocytes. Thus, automation has advanced the state of the art for variability beyond the 400 cell manual differential and well beyond the 200 cell manual differential count. However, it is also noted that considerable differences exist in the analytic variability between different cell types. Using this analysis, analytical variability among the analyzers is least (i.e. best) for eosinophils, slightly larger for lymphocytes and basophils, somewhat larger for neutrophils and largest for monocytes.

Table 5.13 Comparison of duplicate imprecision to total analytic variability on the same sample set*

Parameter	Within-run imprecision CV %	Total variability CV %	Total CV % over precision CV %
Neut (%)	1.13	3.14	2.77
Lymph (%)	2.82	10.1	3.58
Mono (%)	7.70	26.01	3.37
Eos (%)	12.86	26.32	2.00
Baso (%)	55.93	40.96	0.7
Neut (Abs)	2.01	4.96	2.46
Lymph (Abs)	5.51	12.4	2.25
Mono (Abs)	8.76	26.01	2.96
Eos (Abs)	14.00	28.73	2.05
Baso (Abs)	42.8	41.92	0.97

*Approx. 500 samples.

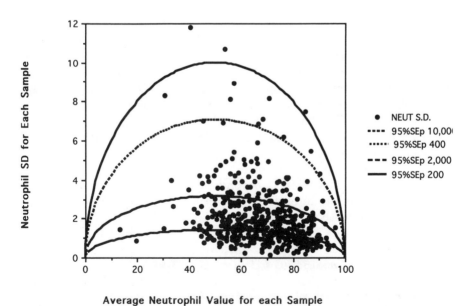

Figure 5.12 Distribution of analytic variability of neutrophils

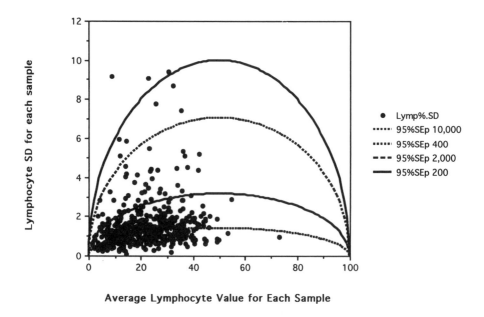

Figure 5.13   Distribution of analytic variability of lymphocytes

This confirms the lack of good correlation results generally reported when monocyte counts are compared to visual differentials. However, the variability among analyzers for monocytes is still within the 400 cell level, begins to drop below 95% at 600 cells and only falls below 90% at 800 cells. The basophil variability seems contained within the boundary of 2000 cell sampling error. Thus, it is still not clear whether the poor correlation results which are generally reported for basophils are determined by sampling error or method issues. However, it is clear that resolution of this issue is beyond the ability to measure through the use of a 400 cell differential as prescribed by H20-A (NCCLS, 1992) for the reference method.

ASSESSING CLINICAL SENSITIVITY

One important feature of the performance of a multiparameter cell counter is the ability to flag specimens which require additional testing. Since modern hematology analyzers do not complete the traditional

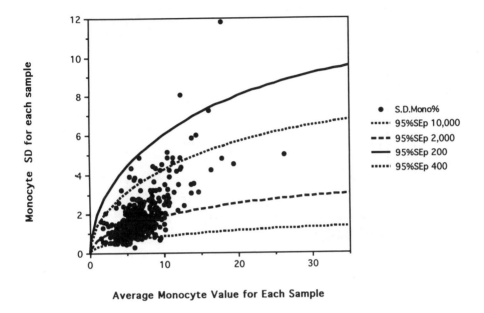

Figure 5.14 Distribution of analytic variability of monocytes

analysis of abnormal cells and abnormal morphology those specimens containing these clinically significant results must be referred to a microscopist. In addition, multiparameter cell counters generally have a set of internal and customer selected alarms which warn the user of suspect results requiring confirmation. Performance of the system specifically with regard to flagging abnormal specimens is generally termed *clinical sensitivity*.

Performance of the system regarding clinical sensitivity is established with respect to a microscopic evaluation of the peripheral blood film in terms of: agreement, false positive and false negatives. Obviously, the ideal situation is 100% agreement with no false flags at all. In that case, the concern is only how many samples require additional work-up and how to efficiently organize the total workload of the hematology laboratory (the subject of the following chapter). However, the ideal case is not yet achieved with any modern instrument. Thus, one important aspect of the total performance of modern cell counting systems is the determination of clinical sensitivity and the numerical values for both false positive and false negative rates.

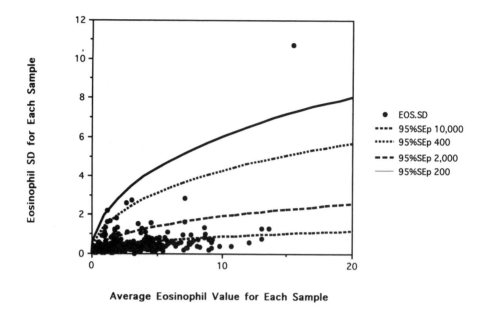

Figure 5.15 Distribution of analytic variability of eosinophils

The following sections will discuss the protocols by which clinical sensitivity is measured and the results obtained with current systems.

PROTOCOLS FOR EVALUATING CLINICAL SENSITIVITY

The goal of a measurement of clinical sensitivity is to show how well a particular cell counting system can identify abnormalities for further study by human observers or by other follow-up testing and to compare this ability to the system in routine use. To perform a clinical sensitivity study there are three separate activities which have to be conducted: first, one must develop reference or normal value ranges for both the test and the reference method; second, one must determine the sensitivity to finding abnormal samples for both methods; and third, one must arbitrate the results when reference and test methods disagree.

As with the studies of clinical accuracy, protocols for assessing clinical sensitivity have been developed providing uniform procedures and the ability to compare data. The method described below follows the NCCLS procedure published as H20-A (NCCLS, 1992). The protocol is shown schematically in Figure 5.17 and consists of three phases:

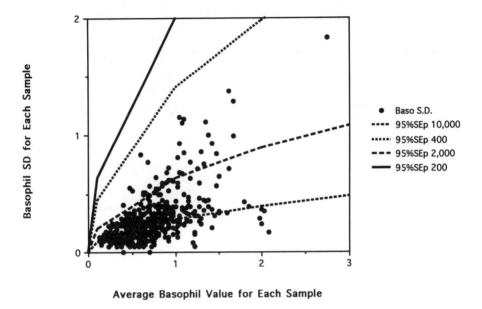

Figure 5.16 Distribution of analytic variability of basophils

Table 5.14 Percentage of specimens with analytic variability within range of expected sampling variability at different numbers of cells counted

Cell type	200 cell	400 cell	600 cell	800 cell	1000 cell	1500 cell	2000 cell	10 000 cell
Neut (%)	99.4	97.0	97.0	94.2	92.5	87.1	81.0	31.2
Lymph (%)	99.4	98.1	96.9	95.2	94.1	91.4	87.4	35.1
Mono (%)	99.3	95.8	91.7	86.5	81.0	67.3	54.1	1.8
Eos (%)	99.6	98.7	98.3	97.2	96.9	95.2	93.4	59.3
Baso (%)	100	100	99.2	98.0	97.6	93.9	89.6	36.9

1. Establishing reference (or normal) ranges.
2. Determining the sensitivity and specificity for flagging abnormal specimens.
3. Arbitration of discrepancies.

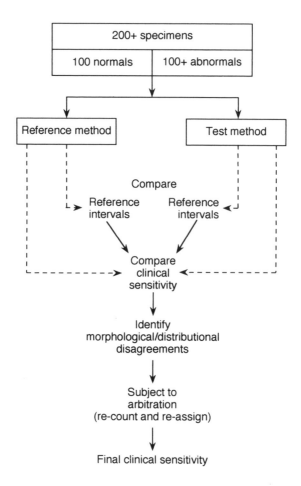

Figure 5.17 Outline of experimental protocol. From NCCLS (1992) with permission

Establishing normal ranges

A minimum of 100 normal individuals are generally used for this part of the study. While it is recognized that a definition of normal is controversial, for the purposes of this protocol, normal means an individual who has:

- No clinical evidence of a medical disorder known to affect the differential leukocyte count.
- No episodes of upper respiratory infection.

- A blood count within the reference range for all of the elements of the complete blood count including the total leukocyte count.
- Serum chemistry values if available that are not grossly abnormal.

Individuals may qualify as normal if they fulfill the above criteria, are laboratory personnel, outpatients coming for periodic check-ups, or patients admitted for elective procedures. Blood donors are satisfactory normals if the sample is taken before the donation (post-donation samples may be altered). The normal samples are used to define the reference ranges for both the instrument under test and the method in routine use. The procedure is as follows:

Step 1

A histogram is constructed for each parameter from the normal values initially obtained.

Step 2

These histograms are then studied and any outlier results eliminated.

Step 3

From the histograms a reference range of values is established for each parameter. The reference range is defined non-parametrically as the central 95% of the normal population. Therefore, with 100 samples, exclude the highest and lowest two values for a total of four for each parameter of this system.

Step 4

Tabulate these reference ranges for each method: the test method; and the method in routine use.

Determining sensitivity for finding abnormal samples

Samples for testing clinical sensitivity should be selected from the entire laboratory workload over a minimum of a two week period. In general, the larger the sample series, the greater the confidence in the results. Samples should include all types of samples typically analyzed in the laboratory. In addition, the test method should be challenged against the most severe abnormalities the laboratory may encounter. To accomplish this it may be necessary to search out specific abnormal cases, process them by both methods then insert them at random as test samples. A list of specific sample types which should be included is given in Table 5.15.

Table 5.15 Specimen types to be included in clinical sensitivity study

Clinical condition	Characteristic leukocyte differential count finding	Absolute cell count	Proportional cell count* (%)
Acute inflammation Bacterial infection	Granulocytosis and/or	$\geqslant 9.0 \times 10^9/l$	> 80
	Left shift† (band-forms)	$\geqslant 0.9 \times 10^9/l$	> 6
Chronic inflammation	Monocytosis	$\geqslant 0.8 \times 10^9/l$	> 10
Parasitic infection Allergic reaction	Eosinophilia	$\geqslant 0.5 \times 10^9/l$	> 7
Viral infections infectious mononucleosis cytomegalovirus infection infectious hepatitis	Lymphocytosis and/or Lymphocytes, variant forms†	$\geqslant 3.5 \times 10^9/l$ $\geqslant 0.7 \times 10^9/l$	> 50
Aplastic anemia, chemotherapy	Granulocytopenia	$\leqslant 1.5 \times 10^9/l$	< 10
HIV infection	Lymphopenia	$\leqslant 1.0 \times 10^9/l$	< 7
Acute leukemia	Immature cells, including blasts†	$\geqslant 0.1 \times 10^9/l$	> 2
Severe anemia myelophthisic anemia	Nucleated red blood cells†	$\geqslant 0.02 \times 10^9/l$	> 2

*In addition to noted absolute counts, the specimens should also have these proportional counts.
†Findings for morphological classification; other findings are considered to be distributional changes. Aim to include at least five cases of each condition in the clinical sensitivity study.
Reproduced with permission from H20-A, *Reference Leukocyte Differential Count (Proportional) and Evaluation of Instrumental Methods; Approved Standard*, NCCLS, 771 E. Lancaster Avenue, Villanova, PA 19085, USA

The results are then analyzed as follows:

Step 1

Classify each study sample into normal or abnormal for both the test and the routine method.

Step 2

Subdivide the abnormal cases as follows: those with abnormal proportions of one or more cell types (distributional or quantitative abnormals), using the reference intervals; and those containing abnormal cells (morphological or qualitative abnormals). A study case may have both a distributional and a morphological abnormality. If the cell

Table 5.16   Preliminary morphological classification

		Results of test method	
		Positive (abnormal)	Negative (normal)
Reference method	Positive (abnormal)	TP (true positive)	FN (false negative)
	Negative (normal)	FP (false positive)	TN (true negative)

Summary

Agreement $\quad = \dfrac{TP + TN}{TP + FN + FP + TN} \times 100 = \%$

False positive ratio $\quad = \dfrac{FP}{FP + TN} \times 100 = \%$

False negative ratio $\quad = \dfrac{FN}{FN + TP} \times 100 = \%$

Reproduced with permission from H20-A, *Reference Leukocyte Differential Count (Proportional) and Evaluation of Instrumental Methods; Approved Standard*, NCCLS, 771 E. Lancaster Avenue, Villanova, PA 19085, USA

counter has failed to give differential count results on a particular sample, then exclude that sample from distributional analysis while including it as a morphological abnormality. Keep a list of all samples excluded from distributional analysis.

Step 3

Prepare two matrix tables (distributional and morphological) which summarize these preliminary classifications. Tables 5.16 and 5.17 demonstrate these tables.

Step 4

Prepare a listing of all specimens showing a disagreement. The results of this procedure may be summarized into two categories: samples are in agreement, either as normal or abnormal, and samples showing disagreement.

Arbitrating discrepancies

Arbitration is limited to those samples showing disagreement between the test method and the routine method for either distributional or

Table 5.17   Preliminary distributional classification

		Results of test method	
		Positive (abnormal)	Negative (normal)
Reference method	Positive (abnormal)	TP (true positive)	FN (false negative)
	Negative (normal)	FP (false positive)	TN (true negative)

Summary

Agreement $\quad=\quad\dfrac{\text{TP} + \text{TN}}{\text{TP} + \text{FN} + \text{FP} + \text{TN}}\quad\times\ 100 = \%$

False positive ratio $\quad=\quad\dfrac{\text{FP}}{\text{FP} + \text{TN}}\quad\times\ 100 = \%$

False negative ratio $\quad=\quad\dfrac{\text{FN}}{\text{FN} + \text{TP}}\quad\times\ 100 = \%$

Reproduced with permission from H20-A, *Reference Leukocyte Differential Count (Proportional) and Evaluation of Instrumental Methods; Approved Standard*, NCCLS, 771 E. Lancaster Avenue, Villanova, PA 19085, USA

morphological findings. Arbitration is performed by a qualified examiner with additional expertise and experience using the reference method. The arbitrator must not have performed any of the original counts in this study.

For each sample to be arbitrated first check that the results are valid and that there are no transcription errors. For morphological disagreements check the analyzer results to confirm that no morphological flags were triggered. For distributional disagreements review the duplicate analyses by the reference method and by the test method for each sample to determine whether the difference between duplicate results for each analysis was greater than would be expected due to imprecision of the method using the approach given in the comparability testing section.

At the conclusion of the arbitration step revise the tables of classifications using the arbitration findings to obtain a final distribution of classifications. The results should have now reduced each specimen into either an agreement result, a false/positive, or a false/negative.

Calculate the percentage of agreement, the false/positive ratio, and the false/negative ratio as shown in Table 5.18.

Table 5.18 Clinical sensitivity results. Final classification (from NCCLS, 1992 with permission)

		Test method		
		Positive	Negative	
Reference method	Positive	True positive	False negative	TP + FN
	Negative	False positive	True negative	TN + FP
		TP + FP	TN + FN	TP + TN + FP + FN

Agreement = TP + TN/TP + TN + FP + FN
(also called "efficiency")
Sensitivity = TP/TP + FN
False positive ratio = FP/TN + FP
Specificity = TN/TN + FP
False negative ratio = FN/TP + FN
Predictive value positive = TP/TP + FP
Predictive value negative = TN/TN + FN

PERFORMANCE EVALUATIONS

Results have now been reported following protocols similar to the one described above for systems from each of the major manufacturers of modern multiparameter cell counters. However, as with the other performance parameters, most of these studies considered the performance of an individual system in a particular laboratory. Since the results of flagging studies are highly dependent on the selected sample set and involve subjective analysis using the microscope, comparisons between reports are virtually impossible. Further, there is no credible way to smooth the data by averaging. Fortunately, in recent reports there are some opportunities to select and analyze the data in a meaningful way when side-by-side studies were performed or identical protocols were used in sequential evaluations at the same laboratory. For this purpose we have concentrated on the following data sets:

1. Bentley has reported on clinical sensitivity tests with each of five systems. Four were analyzed in parallel while the fifth was analyzed using identical protocols and similar samples (Bentley et al., 1993, 1994).
2. Buttarello et al. (1993) have reported on the parallel evaluation of four analyzers.
3. Simson and Groner (1995a) have evaluated four systems in parallel.

Table 5.19 Summary results clinical sensitivity: Coulter STKS system

Category	Bentley *et al.* (1993)	Buttarello *et al.* (1993)	Simson and Groner (1995b)
I. Flagging total abnormality*			
% Abnormal	56	62	81
% Agreement	71	86	86
% False positive	12	5	11
% False negative	17	9	2
II. Flagging qualitative abnormality*			
% Abnormal	39	42	49
% Agreement	69	83	74
% False positive	15	6	10
% False negative	15	11	15

*Expressed as a percentage of the total number of samples.

General flagging for abnormal specimens

Tables 5.19 to 5.23 summarize the findings reported in the studies cited above with regard to the agreement between each of the instruments and visual microscopy to detect abnormal specimens. In the first part of each table the total flagging is considered. In this case both distributional and morphological abnormals are included. It is seen in the tables that the performance of the various instruments is similar with agreement of approximately (70%) in separating normal from abnormal.

In the second part of each table the ability to detect the presence of a qualitatively abnormal specimen is considered. This is a more relevant measurement since it determines which specimens will require visual analysis to complete the laboratory report. The results again show a great deal of similarity between instruments. Approximately, equal numbers of false positive and false negative results (approximately 10% each) are noted for each of the instruments studied.

Specific flagging

Each of the modern cell counting systems attempts to break down the abnormal qualitative flags into specific categories such as immature granulocytes, variant lymphocytes, blast cells, etc. Reported data on the performance of these flags is spurious with insufficient studies to demonstrate accurately the performance of the specific flags. Further, as we shall discuss in the next chapter, the abnormal flags for specific types of nucleated cells may have little impact on the operation of the laboratory or the integration of the systems into the laboratory work-

Table 5.20 Summary results clinical sensitivity: Sysmex NE-8000

Category	Bentley et al. (1993)	Buttarello et al. (1993)	Simson and Groner (1995b)
I. Flagging total abnormality*			
% Abnormal	56	62	81
% Agreement	69	86	90
% False positive	13	8	7
% False negative	18	6	3
II. Flagging qualitative abnormality*			
% Abnormal	39	42	49
% Agreement	68	92	67
% False positive	10	2	10
% False negative	22	6	23

*Expressed as a percentage of the total number of samples.

Table 5.21 Summary results clinical sensitivity: Technicon H*1 system

Category	Bentley et al. (1993)	Buttarello et al. (1993)	Simson and Groner (1995b)
I. Flagging total abnormality*			
% Abnormal	56	62	81
% Agreement	68	83	87
% False positive	16	7	9
% False negative	16	10	4
II. Flagging qualitative abnormality*			
% Abnormal	39	42	49
% Agreement	62	86	62
% False positive	20	6	20
% False negative	18	8	18

*Expressed as a percentage of the total number of samples.

flow unless the predictive value for the flag is so high that it can be used as a positive finding without confirmation. This is, unfortunately, not the case for any of the modern cell counting systems.

Specific categories for flagging of abnormal nucleated cells generally include: blast cells, immature granulocytes, elevated band cells, variant lymphocytes, and nucleated red blood cells. Specific flagging for these cell types has been reported by Buttarello (1993) in his comparison of four analyzers, and similarly in the comparison study performed at Long Island Jewish Medical Center. In addition, Bentley has studied specific flagging in his evaluation of the Roche system. Results of these

Table 5.22 Summary results clinical sensitivity: Cell-Dyn 3000 system ⋄

Category	Bentley et al. (1993)	Buttarello et al. (1993)	Simson and Groner (1995b)
I. Flagging total abnormality*			
% Abnormal	56	62	81
% Agreement	70	88	90
% False positive	15	6	4
% False negative	15	6	6
II. Flagging qualitative abnormality*			
% Abnormal	39	42	49
% Agreement	63	82	71
% False positive	18	8	14
% False negative	18	10	15

*Expressed as a percentage of the total number of samples.

Table 5.23 Summary results clinical sensitivity: COBAS HELIOS analyzer

Category	Bentley et al. (1994)	Buttarello et al. (1993)	Simson and Groner (1995b)
I. Flagging total abnormality*			
% Abnormal	61	N/A	N/A
% Agreement	80	N/A	N/A
% False positive	11	N/A	N/A
% False negative	9	N/A	N/A
II. Flagging qualitative abnormality*			
% Abnormal	43	N/A	N/A
% Agreement	75	N/A	N/A
% False positive	17	N/A	N/A
% False negative	8	N/A	N/A

*Expressed as a percentage of the total number of samples.

studies regarding the predictive value of a positive result are presented in Table 5.24. It is seen from this table that for no abnormal cell category are the specific flagging results sufficiently predictive to be used as a positive finding without confirmation. In fact, specific flagging for some categories such as nucleated red blood cells, is generally poor.

State of the art for clinical sensitivity

Determination of the state of the art for clinical sensitivity cannot be done by following the example used in evaluating analytic performance.

Table 5.24 Specific flagging of modern cell counters: predictive value of a specific flag

Flagging category	H*1		STKS		NE-8000		CD-3000		HELIOS
	Ref. 1	Ref. 2	Ref. 1	Ref. 2	Ref. 1	Ref. 2	Ref. 1	Ref. 2	Ref. 3
Immature granulocytes (%)	70	30	69	30	63	47	61	63	28
Blasts (%)	55	23	53	19	75	35	N/A	11	12
Variant lymphocytes (%)	68	37	50	32	37	32	N/A	13	19
NRBC (%)	27	9	67	17	25	25	100	15	47

Ref. 1: Buttarello *et al.* (1993).
Ref. 2: Simson and Groner (1995b).
Ref. 3: Bentley *et al.* (1994).

The test of clinical sensitivity only exists as a result of the inability of modern cell counters to classify abnormal samples. Consequently, the measurement of performance is determined solely by the percentage of agreement and the actual number of false positive and false negative results. These results will, of course, be dependent on the nature of the sample set. In laboratories processing large numbers of normal specimens concern is predominantly for false negative results, while in laboratories processing a large number of abnormal specimens concern is also for false positive results.

At first glance the presence of the high numbers of disagreements seen in Tables 5.19–5.23 is alarming. However, to put this in perspective one must consider two points:

- First, what was the nature of the false negatives? That is, what were the qualitative abnormalities that were missed?
- Second, how do these results compare to what would be expected in routine visual microscopy? That is, how well would typical microscopists perform if challenged with the same protocol?

Review of the results reported by Buttarello, as well as those obtained in the study at LIJ Medical Center, shows that the false negative results are principally accounted for by specimens containing either variant lymphocytes (6–10%) or an elevated band cell count. This is illustrated in Table 5.25, where the details of the specimens which were missed in each study are indicated.

Koepke has studied and reported (Koepke *et al.*, 1985) on the performance of typical microscopists in flagging abnormal specimens. In these

Table 5.25 Analysis of false negative flags for qualitative abnormality

Flagging category	H*1		STKS		NE-8000		CD-3000		HELIOS
	Ref. 1	Ref. 2	Ref. 1	Ref. 2	Ref. 1	Ref. 2	Ref. 1	Ref. 2	Ref. 3
Immature granulocytes	0		1		1		2		4
Blasts	0		0		1		0		0
Variant lymphocytes	2		2		3		0		4
NRBC	0		0		0		0		11
Total (% of abnormal)	6		6		10		4		16

Ref. 1: Buttarello *et al.* (1993).
Ref. 2: Simson and Groner (1995).
Ref. 3: Bentley *et al.* (1994).

Table 5.26 Flagging performance: comparison of instrument results to 100 cell manual results

Category*	Instruments range (from Tables 5.19–23)	Manual (Koepke *et al.* 1985)
I. Flagging total abnormality		
% Abnormal	56–62	85
% Agreement	68–88	80
% False positive	5–16	2
% False negative	6–16	18
II. Flagging qualitative abnormality		
% Abnormal	39–43	34
% Agreement	62–92	93
% False positive	2–20	0
% False negative	6–22	7

*Expressed as a percentage of the total number of samples.

studies, the H20-A protocol was applied to a hypothetical instrument which consisted of 76 visual microscopists doing a routine 100 cell visual differential. Some pertinent results of this study are reproduced in Table 5.26 where the values obtained by Koepke are compared to those reported in Tables 5.19 to 5.23. As might be expected, the agreement between the routine manual and the reference is greater than that achieved for the automated methods since the manual method in this case is the same method limited primarily by sampling. However, it is also seen from these results that performance of the modern cell counting systems with regard to the flagging of abnormal specimens, in fact, is not substantially worse than the method that they are replacing.

RERERENCES

Bain, B.J. (1989) *Blood Cells—A Practical Guide*, p. 144. Gower Medical Publishing, London.

Bentley, S.A., Johnson, A. and Bishop, C.A. (1993) A parallel evaluation of four automated hematology analyzers. *Am. J. Clin. Pathol.* **100**(6): 626–32.

Bentley, S.A. *et al.* (1994) Flow cytochemical differential leukocyte analysis with quantitation of neutrophil left shift, an evaluation of the COBAS-HELIOS analyzer. *Am. J. Clin. Pathol.* **102**: 223.

Buttarello, M., Gadotti, M., Lorenz, C., Toffalori, E., Ceschini, N., Valentini, A. and Rizzotti, P. (1992) Evaluation of four automated hematology analyzers. A comparative study of differential counts (imprecision and inaccuracy). *Am. J. Clin. Pathol.* **97**(3): 345–52.

Buttarello, M. *et al.* (1993) Diagnostic performance of four automated hematology analyzers. *Am. J. Clin. Pathol.* **100**: 626–32.

Cotlove, E., Harris, E.K. and Williams, G.Z. (1970) Biological and analytic components of variation in long term studies of serum constituents in normal subjects. *Clin. Chem.* **16**: 1028.

Dot, D., Miro, J. and Fuentes-Arderiu (1992) Within-subject biological variation of hematological quantities and analytical goals. *Arch. Pathol. Lab. Med.* **116**: 825.

Elevitch, F.R. (ed.) (1976) College of American Pathologists Conference Report. Conference on Analytical Goals in Clinical Chemistry, at Aspen, Colorado. Skokie, IL, CAP.

Fraser, C.G. (1987) Desirable Standards for hematology tests: a proposal. *Am. J. Clin. Pathol.* **88**: 667.

Fraser, C.G. and Petersen, P.H. (1993) Desirable standards for laboratory tests if they are to fulfill medical needs. *Clin. Chem.* **39**: 1447.

Fraser, C.G., Wilkinson, S.P., Neville, R.G., Knox, J.D.E., King, J.F. and Mac-Walter, R.S. (1989) Biologic variation of common hematologic laboratory quantities in the elderly. *Am. J. Clin. Pathol.* **92**: 465.

Harris, E.K. (1979) Statistical principles underlying analytic goal-setting in clinical chemistry. *Am. J. Clin. Pathol.* **72**: 374.

ICSH (1984) Protocol for evaluation of automated blood cell counters. *Clin. Lab. Haematol.* **6**: 69–84.

ICSH (1994) Guidelines for the evaluation of blood cell analysers including those used for differential leucocyte and reticulocyte counting and cell marker applications. *Clin Lab. Haemat.* **16**: 157–174.

Koepke, J., Dotson, M.A. and Shifman, M.A. (1985) A critical evaluation of the manual/visual differential leukocyte counting method. *Blood Cells* **11**: 173–86.

NCCLS (1982a) *Tentative Guideline EP3-T: Establishing Performance Claims for Clinical Chemical Methods, Replication Experiment.* NCCLS, Villanova, PA 19085, USA.

NCCLS (1982b) *Tentative Guideline EP2-T: Establishing Performance Claims for Clinical Methods, Introduction and Performance Check Experiment.* NCCLS, Villanova, PA 19085, USA.

NCCLS (1982c) *Tentative Guideline EP4-T: Establishing Performance Claims for Clinical Chemical Methods Experiment.* NCCLS, Villanova, PA 19085, USA.

NCCLS (1984) *Tentative Guideline EP5-T: User Evaluation of Precision Performance of Clinical Chemistry Devices*. NCCLS, Villanova, PA 19085, USA.

NCCLS (1989) *Performance Goals for the Internal Quality Control of Multichannel Hematology Analyzers: Proposed Standard*, NCCLS Document H26-P, NCCLS, Villanova, PA 19085, USA.

NCCLS (1992) *Reference Leukocyte Differential Count (Proportional) and Evaluation of Instrumental Methods; Approved Standard*, NCCLS Document H20-A. NCCLS, Villanova, PA 19085, USA.

Rose, M.S. (1971) Epitaph for the MCHC. *Br. J. Med.* **4**: 169.

Ross, D.W., Ayscue, L., Watson, J. and Bentley, S.A. (1988) Stability of hematologic parameters in healthy subjects: intraindividual versus interindividual variation. *Am. J. Clin. Pathol.* **90**: 262.

Rumke, C.L. (1978) The statistically expected variability in differential leukocyte counting. In Koepke, J.A. (ed.) *Differential Leukocyte Counting*. College of American Pathologists, Skokie, IL.

Simson, E. and Groner, W. (1995a) The state of the art for the automation of the WBC differential. Part I: Analytic performance. *Lab. Hematol.* **1**:1.

Simson, E. and Groner, W. (1995b) State of the art for the automated differential. Part II: Clinical Sensitivity. *Lab. Hematol.* **1**: in preparation.

Statland, B.E., Winkel, P., Harris, S.C., Burdsall, M.J. and Saunders, A.M. (1977) Evaluation of biologic sources of variation of leukocyte counts and other hematologic quantities using very precise automated analyzers. *Am. J. Clin. Pathol.* **69**: 48.

Tonks, D.B. (1963) A study of the accuracy and precision of clinical chemistry determinations in 170 Canadian laboratories. *Clin. Chem.* **9**: 217.

Winkel, P., Statland, B.E., Saunders, A.M., Osborn, H. and Kupperman, H. (1981) Within-day physiologic variation of leukocyte types in healthy subjects as assayed by two automated leukocyte differential analyzers. *Am. J. Clin. Pathol.* **75**: 693.

FURTHER READING

Bas, B.M., Catsberg, M.J. and op-de-Kamp, S.L. (1993) A short evaluation of a new haematological analyser: the Cobas Argos 5 Diff. *Eur. J. Clin. Chem. Clin. Biochem.* **31**(9): 603–8.

Brigden, M.L., Page, N.E. and Graydon, C. (1993) Evaluation of the Sysmex NE-8000. Automated hematology analyzer in a high-volume outpatient laboratory. *Am. J. Clin. Pathol.* **100**(6): 618–25.

Broughton, P.M.G., Gowenlock, A.N., McCormak, J.J. and Neill, D.W. (1974) A revised scheme for the evaluation of automated instruments for use in clinical chemistry. *Ann. Clin. Biochem.* **11**: 207–213.

Cohen, A.J., Peerschke, E.I. and Steigbigel, R.T. (1993) A comparison of the Coulter STKS, Coulter S+IV, and manual analysis of white blood cell differential counts in a human immunodeficiency virus-infected population. *Am. J. Clin. Pathol.* **100**(6): 611–17.

Cornbleet, P.J., Myrick, D. and Levy, R. (1993) Evaluation of the Coulter STKS five-part differential. *Am. J. Clin. Pathol.* **99**(1): 72–81.

Cornbleet, P.J. *et al.* (1992) Evaluation of the Cell-Dyn 3000 Differential. *Am. J. Clin. Pathol.* **98**: 603.

Devreese, K., De-Logi, E., Francart, C., Heyndrickx, B., Philippe, J. and Leroux-Roels, G. (1991) Evaluation of the automated haematology analyser Sysmex NE-8000. *Eur. J. Clin. Chem. Clin. Biochem.* **29**(5): 339–45.

d'Onofrio, G., Salvati, A.M., Berti, P. *et al.* (1991) Analysis of leukocyte populations with the Coulter S-Plus STKR as a screening tool for haematological
abnormalities. *Clin. Lab. Haematol.* **13**(1): 51–66.

Drayson, R.A., Hamilton, M.S. and England, J.M. (1992) A comparison of differential white cell counting on the Coulter VCS and the Technicon H1
using simple and multiple regression analysis. *Clin. Lab. Haematol.* **14**(4):
293–305.

England, J.M. (1986) Internal quality control and calibration. In Rowan,
R.M. and England, J.M. (eds.) *Automation and Quality Assurance in
Hematology*. Blackwell Scientific Publications.

England, J.M. and Van Assendelft, O.W. (1986) Automated blood counters and
their evaluation. In Rowan, R.M. and England J.M. (eds.) *Automation and
Quality Assurance in Hematology*. Blackwell Scientific Publications, Oxford.

Fraser, C.G. (1988) The application of theoretical goals based on biological variation data in proficiency testing. *Am. J. Clin. Pathol.* **112**: 404.

Laharrague, P.F., Fillola, G. and Corberand, J.X. (1992) Evaluation of a new
haematology analyser for whole blood counts and full differential (NE-8000).
Nouv. Rev. Fr. Haemat. **34**: 303.

McGrath, C.R., Hitchcock, D.C. and van Assendelft, O.W. (1982) Total White
Blood Cell Counts for Persons Ages 1–74 years with Differential Leukocyte
Counts for Adults Ages 25–74 years. Vital and Health Statistics, Ser 11, No.
220. DHHS Publication No. (PHS) 82–1670. Washington, DC. US Government Printing Office.

Patterson, K.G. and Carter, A.B. (1991) Automated differential counting. *Blood
Rev.* **5**(2): 78–83.

Reardon, D.M., Hutchinson, D., Preston, F.E., and Trowbridge, E.A. (1985) The
routine measurement of platelet volume: a comparison of aperture-impedance
and flow cytometric systems. *Clin. Lab. Haematol.* **7**: 251–7.

Robertson, E.P., Pollock, A., Yau, K.S. and Chan, L.C. (1992a) Use of technicon
H*1 technology in routine thalassaemia screening. *Med. Lab. Sci.* **49**(4): 259–
264.

Robertson, E.P., Lai, H.W. and Wei, D.C. (1992b) An evaluation of leucocyte
analysis on the Coulter STKS. *Clin. Lab. Haematol.* **14**(1): 53–68.

Rowan, R.M. and Fraser, C. (1982) Platelet size distribution analysis. In van
Assendelft, O.W. and England, J.M. (eds.) *Advances in Hematological
Methods: the Blood Count*, pp. 125–41. CRC Press, Boca Raton.

Salvati, A.M., d'Onofrio, G., Berti, P. *et al.* (1991) An assessment of the operating characteristics of Coulter Counter Model S-Plus STKR. *Haematologica*
76(2): 94–103.

Sandberg, S., Thue, G., Christensen, N.G., Lund, P.K. and Rynning, M. (1991)
Performance of cell counters in primary health care. *Scand. J. Prim. Health
Care* **9**(2): 129–33.

Shinton, N.K., England, J.M. and Kennedy, D.A. (1982) Guidelines for the
evaluation of instruments used in haematology laboratories. *J. Clin. Pathol.*
35: 1095–102.

Swaim, W.R. (1991) Laboratory and clinical evaluation of white blood cell differential counts. Comparison of the Coulter VCS, Technicon H-1, and 800-cell
manual method. *Am. J. Clin. Pathol.* **95**(3): 381–8.

Tatsumi, N., Tsuda, I., Funahara, Y., Matsumoto, H., Bunyaratvej, A., Sir-
itanakul, N. and Fucharoen, S. (1992) Size distribution curves of blood cells in
thalassemias and hemoglobin H diseases. *Southeast. Asian. J. Trop. Med.
Public Health* **23** (Suppl 2): 79–85.

Tsakona, C.P., Kinsey, S.E. and Goldstone, A.H. (1992) Use of flow cytochemistry via the H*1 in FAB identification of acute leukaemias. *Acta. Haematol.* **88**(2–3): 72–7.

Turner-Stokes, L., Jones, D., Patterson, K.G., Todd-Pokropek, A., Isenberg, D.A. and Goldstone, A.H. (1991) Measurement of haematological indices of chronic rheumatic disease with two newer generation automated systems, the H1 and H6000 (Technicon). *Ann. Rheum. Dis.* **50**(8): 583–7.

van-Leeuwen, L., Eggels, P.H. and Bullen, J.A. (1991) A short evaluation of a new haematological cell counter—the Cell-Dyn 3000—following a modified tentative NCCLS-procedure. *Eur. J. Clin. Chem. Clin. Biochem.* **29**(2): 105–10.

Verheul, F.E., Spitters, J.M. and Bergmans, C.H. (1993) Evaluation and performance of the Coulter STKS. *Eur. J. Clin. Chem. Clin. Biochem.* **31**(3): 179–86.

Warner, B.A. and Reardon, D.M. (1991) A field evaluation of the Coulter STKS. [see comments]. *Am. J. Clin. Pathol.* **95**(2): 207–17.

Chapter 6

Integrating the Analyzer into the Hematology Laboratory

INTRODUCTION

Several considerations are important in the operation of the hematology laboratory. They are centred upon the provision of accurate and reliable results rapidly enough to be clinically useful, in an efficient and inexpensive manner. We shall consider these factors as we discuss the integration of multiparameter analyzers into the hematology laboratory.

To assure accurate and reliable results, a basic premise of laboratory practice is that quality control results for the batch of patient samples should be within established tolerance limits before results are issued. Patient results are also reviewed to determine whether any are beyond the reportable range of the analyzer for that analyte and to take appropriate steps for re-analysis, e.g. dilution and re-analysis of a sample with a high result.

The total turnaround time for a diagnostic lab report is the time from the writing of the order by the physician to the time the physician receives the results. The eight steps in this process can be summarized as: the physician writes the order; the phlebotomist draws the blood sample; the specimen is transported to the laboratory; the specimen is accessioned and prepared for analysis; the analysis is performed; results are reviewed and verified; the report is transmitted to the requesting physician; and the physician reads the report. From the laboratory viewpoint, turnaround time is often defined as the time from collection of the sample to delivery of the result to the physician; or as the time from receipt of specimen to issuance of report, which is within-laboratory turnaround time. A major consideration in establishing goals for turnaround time is the rapidity with which the physician needs the

Practical Guide to Modern Hematology Analyzers. W. Groner and E. Simson results, e.g. to take care of a critically ill patient as compared with an ambulatory patient having a routine physical examination. An additional consideration for the hematology laboratory is the lability of the specimen.

The hematology laboratory deals with fragile samples. The cells are actively metabolizing and have a limited life in vitro. The only constituent that has any real stability is hemoglobin, as this is measured in any case after hemolysis of the red cells. Platelets swell and then degenerate and neutrophils are the first white cells to degenerate. Red cells swell when kept anaerobically in EDTA and give a falsely higher MCV. Thus, to obtain clinically useful results, the analyses have to be performed within a few hours after the blood has been drawn from the patient.

The opportunity for preservation of the sample is limited and consists virtually only of making fixed stained smears for microscopic examination. Furthermore, for stained smears there is an EDTA effect on the morphology of white cells that makes microscopic recognition of cells in old blood more difficult. Thus the smears themselves have to be made from relatively fresh blood and be fixed within a few hours after specimens have been drawn. The NCCLS in document H20-A (NCCLS, 1992) recommends for the manual reference differential that blood films be prepared within four hours from time of drawing the sample and be stained, or at a minimum, fixed, within one hour of blood film preparation. Automated cell counters provide a benefit in some respects because differential counts can be performed on older blood on most analyzers than manual differential counts on blood films. However, when visual reviews of blood films are then needed to confirm automated differential counts they become more difficult to perform because of the impaired morphology, unless a smear is made at the time of specimen collection and fixed within an hour. Thus for many laboratories, blood films may have to be made on all specimens soon after the blood is received, regardless of whether the laboratory workflow is designed for later visual examination only of specimens whose results have met laboratory criteria for review.

The lability of the specimen, combined with the desire to provide the requesting physician with results as quickly as feasible, make rapidity of operation an important requirement. It is preferable for samples to be analyzed as quickly as possible after receipt. Accumulation of large batches of samples before analysis begins is undesirable. An assembly-line type of operation with few "bottlenecks" is a desirable approach.

Modern multiparameter cell counters have allowed work stations to be consolidated considerably, especially because of the consolidation of the WBC differential with the CBC. The recent history of modern cell counters is essentially consolidation, as more measurements, analyses and calculated values have been added (see Chapter 1). The modern hematology laboratory consists of three to five workstations performing the functions of accessioning, blood film making and staining, manual tests such as sedimentation rates and reticulocytes, the CBC and automated differential workstation, blood film review and manual differentials. This chapter will assess the utility of hematology analyzers in the hematology laboratory and will discuss how to integrate multiparameter analyzers for maximum benefits. In doing so, we shall discuss the factors affecting laboratory operation; we shall examine laboratory workflow and consider how to optimize workflow both within and outside the laboratory; we shall examine criteria for hematologic review and confirmation of analyzer results; and review strategies for internal and external quality control.

FACTORS AFFECTING LABORATORY OPERATION

There are several factors that contribute to delay in analyzing the sample and providing results to the requesting physician. The factors that should be considered can be divided into pre-analytical, analytical and post-analytical.

PRE-ANALYTICAL FACTORS

Pre-analytical factors include the within-laboratory operation as well as circumstances that cause delay in the specimen reaching the laboratory (pre-laboratory factors):

Pre-laboratory factors

These include:

1. Proximity or alternatively distance of the laboratory from the site where blood was drawn; in most cases, the laboratory is some distance from where blood was drawn.
2. Delay between drawing of blood and transport to laboratory, i.e. frequency of specimen tube pick-up from the blood-drawing site.
3. Mode and speed of specimen transport to the laboratory, such as by automated specimen transport system, for example a pneumatic tube; messenger on foot (in a hospital or other facility); automobile, airplane, etc.

Within-laboratory factors

Within-laboratory factors include:

1. Speed with which specimens are accessioned into the laboratory data system, whether manual or a Laboratory Information System.
2. Pre-analytical workflow: Labeling specimens, making and staining blood films, aliquots for manual tests, batching of specimens.

ANALYTICAL FACTORS

Analytical factors that should be considered include:

1. Sampling: is it manual or automated; open-tube or closed-tube?
2. Dwell-time. This is the time the sample is in the analyzer before analysis is performed. This is now typically very short—less than a minute in modern multiparameter analyzers.
3. The cycle time, i.e. the time between sampling successive samples, is now typically 25–40 seconds, i.e. an analysis rate of 100–140 per hour.
4. The review and approval of results, either in batches or as each sample is analyzed.
5. Further analyses, such as repeat analysis, blood film review, a manual differential count, platelet count, etc.

POST-ANALYTICAL FACTORS

1. Final review and approval of results.
2. Transmission of results to physician by courier or mail, facsimile transmission, remote printer, computer terminal, etc.

We shall now discuss these aspects in greater detail.

LABORATORY WORKFLOW

WORKFLOW WITHIN THE LABORATORY

The analytical process consists of all analyses performed on each specimen, both automated and manual. The workflow within the laboratory is organized to optimize speed and efficiency and minimize costs. There is the simultaneous objective of enhancing quality by combining automation and manual operation synergistically; for example, the highly precise automated differential count is combined with the high accuracy of specific cell identification by visual examination of the blood film. In considering the efficiency of the analytical process, all aspects need to considered. For example, if slow, labor intensive and therefore costly microscopy is a large component of the analysis for many specimens, this will have a large impact on the overall speed, efficiency and cost of the analytical process as a whole. Thus, improvements in the speed, efficiency and cost of the automated analyzer may be largely nullified if it increases the requirement for manual analysis of the specimen.

There are several workstations within the hematology laboratory. The work performed in each varies depending on instrumentation and there may be consolidation by some laboratories of tasks into one workstation, whereas other laboratories may perform the same tasks at two separate workstations, depending on workload and the size of the laboratory. Also, depending on the size of the laboratory and the workload it handles, there may be duplication of certain workstations. Sample and information flow between workstations may vary. Optimization of workflow within the laboratory can increase efficiency and reduce costs significantly.

Workstations

The basic workstations are:

1. Accessioning and specimen handling.
2. Blood film preparation and specimen aliquotting.
3. The analyzer workstation (CBC, or CBC and WBC differential; also automated reticulocytes).
4. The microscopy workstation for blood film examination and manual differentials.
5. Manual tests, such as reticulocytes, ESRs (erythrocyte sedimentation rates) and manual platelet counts.

Accessioning and specimen handling

Accessioning consists of receiving the specimens, checking the accuracy and adequacy of specimen labels and the requisition forms, checking sufficiency of specimens; logging specimens and requests into the laboratory record-keeping system, which is either a manual log-book or computer terminal; assigning unique accession numbers for each specimen; assigning priority for processing (stat, urgent or routine); recording tests requested for each specimen and distributing specimens to appropriate workstations.

In some laboratories, direct entry into the hematology analyzer data station serves some of the functions of accessioning. As most modern analyzers read bar-codes, bar-code labels may be printed at the accession station and attached to specimens; the accessioning process is considerably simplified and accelerated if bar-coded labels are attached to specimen tubes at the time of phlebotomy. This is possible in hospitals where test requests are entered into the Hospital Information System, which then generates a bar-coded label containing patient information and requested tests.

Blood film preparation and aliquotting

This is where the specimen is examined for clots, a blood film is made and aliquots are removed for the performance of manual tests, such as sedimentation rates, reticulocytes, and manual platelet counts performed at a separate workstation.

The analyzer workstation

This is where a CBC analyzer or a CBC plus differential analyzer is used to perform the majority of the analyses. In the stat situation, the sample may be brought directly to the CBC analyzer from the accessioning station rather than through the blood film preparation station. In such instances, the sample will then be routed to the blood film and manual station after CBC or CBC plus differential analysis.

Results of the CBC or CBC plus differential analysis need to be reviewed by an operator and then a decision is made as to which specimens will need further analysis for confirmation or validation of the results of the analyzer or whether the analyzer is unable to perform a valid count on one or more of the cell types. This is discussed in more detail later in this chapter under review criteria.

Microscopy workstation

At the microscopy workstation, the blood film is reviewed to confirm abnormalities; to detect and identify abnormalities that have been flagged but not identified; to perform a manual differential when necessary and to make a manual (visual) estimate of platelet count on the blood film for low platelet counts.

The manual workstation

If separate from the blood film station, this is where sedimentation rates, reticulocyte counts and platelet counts may be performed. Analyzers are now available that can either perform a reticulocyte count directly (Sysmex R1000 and flow cytometers) or which have an attach-

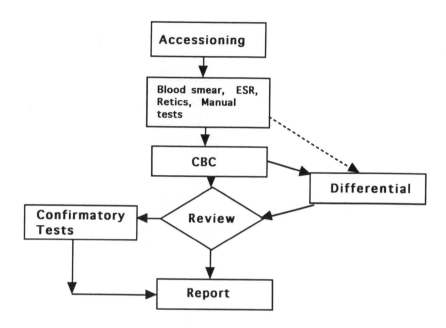

Figure 6.1 Flowchart of automated CBC and manual differential

ment whereby off-line preparation of the sample is performed before analysis on the analyzer (Technicon H*3, Coulter STKS and MAXM and Abbott Cell-Dyne 3500). Thus, for selected samples, the CBC and differential analyzer will perform the reticulocyte count as well.

Workflow Options

Figures 6.1, 6.2, 6.3 and 6.4 give some typical examples of the way the workflow may be handled.

Figure 6.1 is for a laboratory with an automated CBC analyzer, but with manual differentials only. Differentials are performed only when specifically requested by the physician; furthermore, in many laboratories, differentials are not performed unless the WBC count is outside the normal range, even if requested by the physician. Differentials may be performed in parallel with CBCs, but are usually performed after results of the CBC are available, to take advantage of blood film review to confirm abnormalities of CBC results.

Figure 6.2 shows a workflow using a multiparameter analyzer with CBC and five part differential capability. Specimens are accessioned. At the blood film workstation, the tube is opened, checked for clots, smears

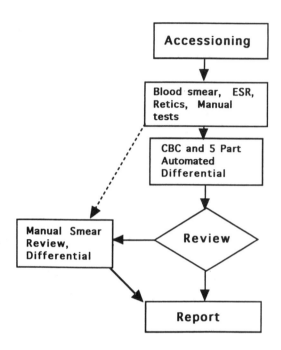

Figure 6.2 Flowchart of CBC and automated five part differential

are made and aliquots taken for manual tests such as ESR and reticu-locytes. The tubes are then re-capped and put into racks for analysis by the cell counter. Analyzer results are reviewed by the operator (or another technologist) to determine whether the analysis should be repeated, whether a blood film has to be examined, a manual differen-tial performed, or whether the report may be issued without further analysis. Criteria used for making these decisions will be discussed in detail later in this chapter.

Figure 6.3 shows a workflow which is driven by the need for rapid turnaround for Stat analyses, but which is applicable to the general workflow of the hematology laboratory. The important difference between this workflow and that shown in Figure 6.2 is that specimens are analyzed before being checked for clots. This approach causes some trepidation, because of the fear that clots may obstruct the analyzer; however, modern analyzers have clot detection systems as well as pro-cedures for rapid washout to remove clots without delaying the analysis process. (Certain specimens, e.g. micro samples from skin puncture, should still be opened and checked for clots before analysis; these usually have to be handfed to the system, so that a different procedure

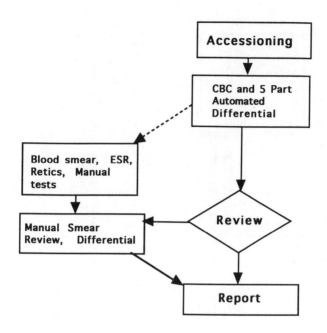

Figure 6.3 Flowchart of STAT CBC and five part differential

is necessary in any case.) Turnaround time is shortened considerably for many specimens, as results can be reported without blood film review. Depending on the laboratory protocol and regulatory requirements, blood films may be made on all specimens, whether examined or not; or only on those which are abnormal and require microscopy. New York State, for example, requires that slides of peripheral blood showing any abnormality be retained for one year; it does not require that smears from blood with normal results be retained.

Figure 6.4 shows a system that automates the workflow shown in Figure 6.3. It has recently been introduced by Sysmex as the HS system (Hayashi, 1992). The system consists of a combination of one or more NE-8000 or SE-9000 CBC and differential analyzers, the SP automatic blood film preparation device, and optionally an R1000 reticulocyte analyzer, connected by a conveyer belt; with a controller to direct each specimen to any of the processing units as specimens pass along the conveyer belt. Specimens are analyzed by the NE-8000 (or SE-9000), which has programmed into it the criteria for manual blood film review or manual differential; a blood film is automatically made at the SP station on any specimen that meets the criteria.

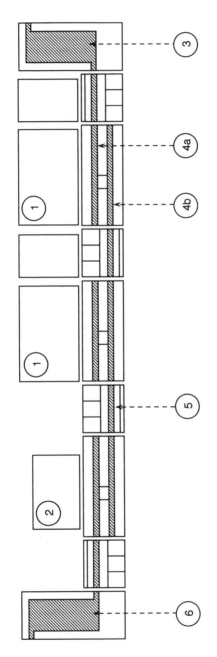

Figure 6.4 Components of the HS-302. Analyzers: 1, NE-8000; 2, SP-1. Transportation system: 3, starting pool unit; 4, conveyor unit, (a) analysis line, (b) bypass line; 5, rack sliding unit; 6, finish pool unit

WORKFLOW OUTSIDE THE LABORATORY

Specimen collection

Specimens are collected by venipuncture, finger prick or heel puncture. There are several excellent texts that deal with the subject in detail and provide guidance on collecting the specimen, safety precautions, labeling, etc. (NCCLS, 1991a, 1991b; Lotspeich-Steininger *et al.*, 1992).

In drawing blood from patients the integrity of the specimen is paramount. For example, aspiration of blood from an indwelling venous or arterial catheter, with resulting contamination with intravenous fluid, must be avoided. Also, the margination of cells and the demargination of cells under certain conditions such as stress has to be considered. Thus in a patient who is extremely nervous or in a child who is crying and agitated at the time of venipuncture, neutrophils and eosinophils may be increased because of cortisone release. Similarly, application of a tourniquet for too long could affect the results obtained.

The safety of the phlebotomist during collection is an important issue which is governed in the United States by regulations from the Occupational Safety and Health (OSHA), recommendations from the Centers for Disease Control (CDC) and NCCLS. The textbooks referred to above and references from NCCLS give details of the precautions that must be taken. Special reference should be made to NCCLS publication M29-T2 (NCCLS, 1991a) for details. Accurate labeling of requisition forms and specimen containers is essential: the texts referred to above give instructions. All applicable regulatory requirements from national, state or other applicable health departments must be followed.

Stability of the specimen

The specimen is a "fragile" specimen with limited stability for the various cellular constituents to be measured. Considerations of stability at room temperature and when the specimen is refrigerated must be kept in mind. In general, room temperature storage is preferable to refrigerated storage for most of the parameters, especially the WBC differential count for all analyzers. The anticoagulant itself (usually EDTA) has an adverse effect over time on the morphology, as well as the analyzer response characteristics of the cells, especially for leukocytes.

Impact of specimen collection, storage and transport on workflow within the laboratory

The number of specimens arriving at the laboratory through the hours it is open is seldom constant. The laboratory has to be staffed and equipped to be able to provide sufficient rapid turn-around-time at peak periods as well as quiet periods. For instance, if the goal for turnaround time is one hour the laboratory specimen throughput capacity (including the analyzer) must exceed the specimen receipt rate at its peak by a comfortable margin. If the laboratory is open 24 hours per day, 7 days a week, it is likely that there will be extended quiet periods during which only stat specimens will be analyzed, less staff can be on duty and throughput of analyzers can be relatively low. However, at peak periods, specimen throughput and analyzer throughput become a major concern. This is driven by three factors: (1) the need to analyze the "fragile" samples within a sufficiently short time; (2) the need to provide results on very ill inpatients rapidly enough to assist physicians managing their care and (3) for ambulatory patients, the need to provide results to physicians rapidly enough to facilitate care as well as meeting competition from other laboratories striving for the same clients.

It is beneficial for the laboratory to be able to smooth out specimen receipt and transport, and even, where possible, specimen collection. Figure 6.5 shows an example from our own laboratory at LIJ. Specimen receipt was monitored during January 1991 and again in March 1991 after some changes were made. During January, from midnight to 7 am a constant low volume of approximately 30 specimens per hour, consisting of "stat" and "urgent" specimens, was received. Phlebotomists began duty at 6 am and drew specimens according to requisitions that had been completed by the time they arrived on each patient unit. The phlebotomists completed their rounds through the patient units in approximately 3 hours. Specimens were brought to the laboratory by messengers as they went on their separate rounds through the patient units. Doctors' rounds begin at 7 am on some units and 8 am on others. Most of the venipunctures resulting from these doctors' rounds were performed by ward personnel amongst their other duties during the morning, because the phlebotomists had already left the units by the time the requisitions were completed. The hourly number of specimens received by the laboratory was approximately 70 between 7 am and 9 am. The number of specimens received between 9 am and 10 am was approximately 110 and between 10 am and 11 am peaked at 140, dropped to 85 between 11 am and 12 noon and 65 the next hour. The bulk of the workload only began to be analyzed a little before noon and results only become available well into the afternoon and into the evening shift, which begins at 4 pm. There was a backlog of specimens in the laboratory waiting for analysis in the late morning and stretching into the afternoon and evening. For the remainder of the day, the number of specimens received by the laboratory averaged approximately 60 per hour till 7 pm and then progressively declined to the night level of 30 per hour. Many technologists who began work at 7 am and 8 am were relatively unproductive for the first 3 hours of their 8 hour shift. A

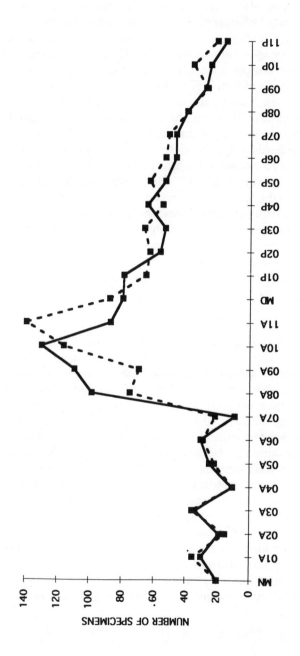

Figure 6.5 Specimen receipt by hour at Long Island Jewish Medical Center. Solid line, 11–15 March 1991; broken line, average for period from November 1990 to February 1991

single multiparameter analyzer coped comfortably with the workload from 8 pm to 7 am. However, even two analyzers, each with an effective throughput speed of 85 specimens per hour could not cope with the peak workload; in addition, as the analyzer differential count was a three part differential, many specimens required fairly extensive manual review.

The relatively simple measure of a second phlebotomy round was implemented on 1 March 1991. Phlebotomists made two successive rounds through the patient units with a short break between them. In addition, coordination between phlebotomist and messenger rounds was improved. The number of specimens received by the laboratory earlier in the day increased to approximately 110/hour between 7 am and 9 am and peaked at 125 between 9 am and 10 am, dropping to 85 between 10 am and 11 am, compared with 140 previously. Although the number of specimens per hour received by the laboratory after 1 pm remained approximately the same, they could be processed much more rapidly, because the backlog from the morning was much less. Turnaround time for the morning specimens improved; the number of stat and urgent requests dropped because the requests from doctors' rounds could be dealt with by the phlebotomists in their regular rounds; and technologists were more productive throughout their shift.

HEMATOLOGIC REVIEW OF ANALYZER RESULTS

In the hematology laboratory, review of patient results reaches a level far beyond that of other laboratories, such as clinical chemistry. There is fairly widespread skepticism of results produced by hematology analyzers, especially for the differential count. Hematological review is defined as the performance of a test or procedure by a person skilled in the art of laboratory hematology to confirm or validate analyzer results or obtain results that the analyzer was unable to produce on that blood sample. This is in contrast to clinical chemistry, where alternative analysis methods are hardly ever employed and action usually consists of re-analysis on the same analyzer without dilution to confirm the result, or with dilution if the result was high. The ideal multiparameter hematology analyzer would require no hematologic review of specimens after analysis, but this goal has not yet been achieved. In most laboratories, a fairly high proportion of samples still require review even when analyzed by the most modern multiparameter hematology analyzers.

REASONS FOR HEMATOLOGIC REVIEW

There are several reasons why hematologic review may be considered necessary. In general, the objective is to reduce the number of samples requiring review to the greatest possible extent, while not endangering the patient by reporting false or misleading results, especially false negative results. A false positive result from an analyzer merely causes additional work for the laboratory; whereas a false negative result might significantly affect the diagnosis and management of a patient.

Reasons for review may be summarized as follows.

White cell differential

1. The analyzer fails to give one or more results for that sample: either there is no result; or there is a result which the analyzer has indicated by an asterisk or some other means may be unreliable.
2. The analyzer identifies or flags the presence of abnormal cells which it is not able to count. The analyzer may or may not flag the specific cell type. These are known as morphological flags.*
3. The number and/or proportion of one or more normal cell types is outside the reference interval for the normal population, or outside review limits established by the laboratory, which are frequently broader than the reference interval.

Red cells

Results produced by the analyzer indicate the need for further analysis on the same sample to provide a more comprehensive report, e.g. detailed review of red cell morphology on a slide for a sample with a low hemoglobin result and abnormal red cell indices; or to confirm a red cell morphology flag produced by the analyzer.

Platelets

To confirm a low platelet count or a platelet morphology flag.

For all cell types

One or more results is significantly different from previous results of that patient and exceeds the "delta check". Delta checks operate to reduce hematological review by recognizing previously detected validated abnormalities. Delta limits should be established by taking into account analyzer imprecision and drift, as well as physiological considerations. Delta limits in use in our hematology laboratory are as

---

*In the United States, performance claims by manufacturers for their analyzers are subject to review by the Food and Drug Administration; at the time of writing, no manufacturer is in a position to make performance claims for counting abnormal cells.

follows: hemoglobin: 2.5 g/dl, hematocrit: 7.5%, MCHC: 1.5 g/dl, MCV: 5.0 fl, WBC: 5.0×10^9/l, neutrophils and other white cell types: 0.1×10^9/l. Note that the delta limits for a differential count are very tight. When a technologist is verifying present results, our Laboratory Information System only displays to the technologist previous results for those analytes which exceed the delta limits. The tight limits for the differential components enable us to detect that a manual differential count has been performed on the patient previously, as we do not repeat manual differential counts within 48 hours. However, the technologist can decide from the displayed result after 48 hours whether in fact the manual differential should be repeated.

Review criteria must be established for each of the cell types based on the reasons listed above. The criteria vary depending on the performance of the analyzer and the characteristics of the analyzer. Manufacturer's literature provides some guidance, but several factors particular to each laboratory have to be considered. Setting valid and appropriate review criteria for the analyzer(s) in use is one of the most important and challenging aspects of integrating a hematology analyzer into the workflow of the hematology laboratory.

FACTORS INFLUENCING REVIEW CRITERIA

The reference range or interval

Because quantitation of normal cell types by modern hematology analyzers is sufficiently accurate and precise, it is unnecessary to review a blood film on samples with only normal cell types, all within the reference intervals and with normal CBC values (Brigden and Page, 1990). Reference intervals (normal ranges) can therefore be used to minimize review. Using the same rationale, review criteria can be set to be much broader than the reference intervals without increasing the risk of false quantitation. For best clinical and operational utility, the reference intervals on which the review criteria are based should be age and sex specific. For example (as can be seen in Table 6.1 on reference intervals for the CBC, and Table 6.2 on reference intervals for the differential), the WBC reference interval and the absolute lymphocyte count reference interval in the first years of life are significantly different from those of adults, so that what may be regarded as highly abnormal for an adult could be normal for an infant at birth or a few months old. Thus adult review criteria would be inappropriate for babies and vice versa.

In setting review criteria for each of the white cell types, levels are also chosen to assist in the prevention of false negative morphological flags (see Chapter 5). For example, as the neutrophil count increases,

Table 6.1 Reference intervals: CBC

Age	WBC × 10⁹/l	Hb (male) g/l	Hb (female) g/l	Hematocrit (male) (%)	Hematocrit (female) (%)	Platelet × 10⁹/l
At birth	9–30	17–23	17–23	50–62	50–62	300–750
1–6 months	8–24	9–18.5	9–18.5	41–54	41–54	300–750
6 months–1 yr	7–20	11–14	11–14	33–42	33–42	300–750
1–4 yrs	6–17.5	9–14	9–14	31–39	31–39	250–600
4–6 yrs	5–15.5	10–15	10–15	32–40	32–40	250–550
6–10 yrs	5–14.5	10–15	10–15	34–42	34–42	250–500
10–21 yrs	4.5–13.5	11–15	11–15	38–46	38–46	200–450
21+ yrs	4–10	14–18	12–16	42–52	36–46	140–450

Table 6.2 Reference intervals: differential in cells × 10⁹/l

Age	Neut	Lymph	Mono	Eos	Baso	NRBC
At birth	1.6–9	2.2–9.8	0.1–1	0–1.4	0–0.3	0–5.4
7 days	2.1–8.0	3.1–8.4	0.2–1.8	0.2–1.9	0–0.3	0–0.1
1–5 yrs	1.5–7.0	2.5–8.5	0.2–1.3	0.1–1.2	0–0.2	0
5–10 yrs	1.8–7.7	1.7–5.5	0.2–1.3	0.1–1.0	0–0.2	0
10–18 yrs	1.5–6.0	1.5–4.0	0.2–1.3	0.1–0.8	0–0.2	0
18+ yrs	2.0–6.5	1.5–3.5	0.2–1.0	0.1–0.5	0–0.2	0

so the probability of immature myeloid cells such as bands, metamyelocytes, myelocytes and promyelocytes in the peripheral blood increases. Criteria for review are set at levels where abnormal cells might be expected, but not necessarily flagged. This has relevance to the discussion below on false negative and false positive flags.

The patient population

Knowledge of patient population characteristics can be used to influence the review criteria. For example: We would expect different results in patients from an anemia clinic or from the oncology floor to those from patients merely having a routine physical examination.

Confidence in analyzer results

The characteristics, capabilities and limitations of the analyzer are important factors which affect the criteria for review. The question of real versus perceived limitations also impacts the setting of criteria. For example: If someone perceives that the analyzer does not provide an accurate neutrophil count outside the normal range, that person's criteria for review would be much tighter than someone who believes that the analyzer's neutrophil count is accurate. In many laboratories with new hematology analyzers, criteria for review become less stringent as confidence in the analyzer's performance builds. To provide guidance to users, much time, effort and money is expended by investigators and the companies which manufacture and sell multiparameter analyzers to establish performance characteristics of each of the analyzers on the market for a variety of abnormalities as well as normal subjects. A number of publications describe these performance characteristics, many based on NCCLS H20-A. See Chapter 5 for details of analyzer performance and for literature references to these publications. This published literature is of some help in setting review criteria for particular analyzers in the individual laboratory.

False positive and false negative flags

Manufacturers have gone to great lengths to improve flagging of individual abnormal cell types and most of the publications on analyzer performance list tables of false positives and false negatives for each abnormal cell type flagged. However, the morphological flagging sensitivity is set by the manufacturer and cannot be changed by the laboratory. Thus, the individual laboratorian who, for example, believes that the analyzer is falsely flagging too many samples as having blasts, or conversely, is missing samples with blasts, must develop criteria apart from the blast flag itself to deal with the situation. One means is to couple the flag with limits on the quantitative cell counts as discussed above for neutrophils.

The questions which must be considered are:

1. Is the system sufficiently reliable for false positives and false negatives?
2. What are the clinical consequences of the false negatives in the specific cases reported?
3. If a flag is too sensitive, i.e. if there are too many false positives, is there a grading which may allow less sensitive criteria to be employed in the individual laboratory? For example, for the Technicon H*1, H*2 and H*3 series of analyzers, which have Left Shift 1, 2 and 3 flags, or the Ig/Band 1 and 2 of the Coulter STKS and MAXM, can a flag such as Left Shift 1 or Ig/Band 1 be ignored?
4. Is the counting of certain cell types of such limited clinical value that flags for that cell type could be ignored? Studies of clinical sensitivity for the manual band count show variable results with most showing that it has low sensitivity and slightly better specificity as an indicator of acute infection or inflammation at any age (Dueholm

et al., 1989; Wasserman *et al.*, 1989; Baron and Fink, 1980; Todd, 1974; Christensen *et al.*, 1981). As with any clinical test, sensitivity and specificity bear a reciprocal relationship to each other, so that the chosen indicator point affects both sensitivity and specificity. For example, a level of 15% bands will have less sensitivity and greater specificity for detecting infection than a level of 5% bands, which has greater sensitivity and less specificity. Some studies suggest that automated counting of neutrophils is superior to counting of bands for detecting acute infection (Marchand *et al.*, 1983; Banez and Bacaling, 1988; Wenz *et al.*, 1987). Several laboratories no longer report bands in the differential count (Dutcher, 1984).

5. Realistically, when a particular abnormal cell type is flagged by an analyzer, does the morphologist reviewing the blood film only search for the particular cell type flagged or for any abnormal cells of whatever type they may be? The morphologist clearly focuses attention on the cell type flagged. However, in most laboratories, the person reviewing the smear is expected to detect any abnormalities present as well as validating the analyzer flag. If this is so, then the efficiency of specific cell flagging may be less important than the overall flagging capability of the analyzer. As described in Chapter 5, data for all hematology analyzers shows a lower false negative rate for overall flagging of abnormal specimens than for specific cell types. In contrast to the general direction being followed presently by manufacturers of hematology analyzers, some people would argue that a flag simply for the presence of abnormal cells of any kind may have sufficient utility for general use.

REVIEW ACTIONS

Because of the combined variability of clinical patient specimen mix in laboratories, the analyzers in use, the needs and desires of different clinicians and the different philosophies of laboratory directors, it is impossible to give specific guidance which can be applied to each analyzer in each laboratory. Some general principles can be given. The following list of actions gives some options for each situation which may arise; one or more of the options may be chosen, or actions which are not listed may be taken, depending on individual preference and the recommendations of the manufacturer of the analyzer. The analyzer in all cases is assumed to be functioning well and with satisfactory quality control results. Thus, any failure to give a result, or the generation of a flag, can be assumed to be sample-specific, rather than a manifestation of an analyzer problem. Obviously, a succession of similar flags will raise the question of a problem with the analyzer, which is addressed differently.

The various scenarios are:

1. The analyzer fails to give one or more results on a sample. The actions depend on which results are missing:
   a. Repeat the analysis on the same analyzer. This confirms the problem and sometimes a simple repeat analysis provides results which are clearly preferable to the first results obtained.
   b. Perform the analysis on a different analyzer, preferably with different technology, if one is available.
   c. Perform a manual test; i.e. a visual differential and blood film review, or platelet count, or spun hematocrit etc.

2. The analyzer provides a morphological flag for an abnormal white cell type (with or without an abnormal distribution of normal cell types), or flags for red cell or platelet morphological abnormalities:
   a. Review the blood film to confirm if the abnormal white cell type/s are present, or perform detailed red cell morphology assessment, or assess platelet size and sufficiency.
   b. Perform a visual differential to quantitate the abnormal cell type/s in proportion to the normal cell types.

3. The result exceeds review limits for distributional abnormalities, without any morphological flags:
   a. Review the blood film, firstly to confirm by impression the abnormal distribution, but more importantly to detect any abnormal cells which may not have been flagged. Remember that criteria for review are set at levels where abnormal cells might be expected, but not necessarily flagged.
   b. Perform an eye differential. It may be asked why proportional abnormalities of white cell types should be reviewed with a visual differential because of the high precision afforded by an analyzer count compared to a visual differential count. Possible reasons include:
      i. Cells may be included which should be counted; i.e. variant lymphocytes, or perhaps bands. As none of the analyzers specifically count variant lymphocytes or bands, they are included in the total neutrophil count and the total lymphocyte count respectively. (There may or may not have been a flag for these cell types.) There is a good argument for doing a 200 cell manual count in such cases to obtain the improved precision of a 200 cell count, rather than a 100 cell count.
      ii. This is another means to detect abnormal cell types which have not been flagged.

LEVELS OF REVIEW:

To assure quality of the entire analytical process, including the manual differential, it is important that levels of review be established (Bull, 1991). The review levels are:

1. Medical technologist. The medical technologist, who must have demonstrated expertise in blood film microscopy, performs the first level of review. Criteria for this initial review will vary depending on the factors discussed above. In general, most laboratories will review blood smears on samples where the analyzer has failed to give a result, or has flagged the presence of abnormal white cells, or has flagged for abnormal red cell morphology, or for abnormal platelet morphology. Criteria for review based on abnormal results of normal cell types varies widely. Blood films are examined and manual differential counts performed as necessary.

2. Supervisor. Every laboratory should have criteria for supervisory review of blood films. The criteria in our hematology laboratory at Long Island Jewish Medical Center are:
   a. All alert values (also known as critical or "panic" values).
   b. Any RBC morphology result of +++ or greater.
   c. Red cell inclusions, sickle cells or other abnormal cells.
   d. Any blasts or promyelocytes.
   e. Myelocytes more than 5%.
      Metamyelocytes more than 5%.
      Bands more than 20%.
      Neutrophils less than 10% or more than 90%.
      Eosinophils more than 20%.
      Basophils more than 3%.
      Nucleated RBCs more than 2% in adults and more than 5% in children.
   f. Any white cell congenital abnormalities.

3. Laboratory director. The laboratory director, as an expert morphologist, should provide the final level of review and confirmation of abnormal findings. In our laboratory, the laboratory director reviews any slide on which the supervisor has questions, doubts or concerns.

STRATEGIES FOR CONFIRMATION AND SUPPLEMENTATION OF ANALYZER RESULTS

Most strategies are designed to minimize the additional work required for confirmation and supplementation of analyzer results. Many laboratories now report normal results directly without hematological review.

Many laboratories perform a manual differential count only if their criteria are met by the results reported by the analyzer, as discussed in detail above. Other laboratories will perform a manual differential if it is specifically listed on the requisition form, or at the physician's request, whether or not the criteria are fulfilled. Charges and payment issues also come into play, as different payment may be received for different procedures, even though the information on the report form is the same.

As hematology analyzers with five part differential capability and perhaps also reticulocyte capability become more widely used, the issue of a "peripheral blood cell examination" where the laboratory decides on how it shall be performed, compared with specific requests for part of the peripheral blood examination, together with specific instructions on how it shall be performed (e.g. manual differential), may become greater.

REPORTING RESULTS

The problems consist of melding manual results with the analyzer results. This has controversial aspects, on which opinions differ. Also, if the abnormality which previously led to a manual review remains, what should be done as a follow-up? What strategy should be used for reporting percentage and absolute differential counts? Is it valid to simply multiply the white cell count by the percentage cell types obtained by the manual differential to obtain an absolute differential?

Format

The format is usually decided by the laboratory and may be governed by the Laboratory Information System format. Cumulative reports in tabular form are frequently used for inpatients to facilitate comparison with recent previous results, whereas for outpatients, single reports are usually issued.

Elements of the report from the analyzer

1. Result obtained for each analyte; for the WBC differential, percentage and absolute counts.
2. Reference interval for each analyte (preferably age and sex specific).
3. Indication of an abnormal result (H, L, * etc.), based on age and gender-specific reference intervals.
4. Indication of significant change from previous result (delta).
5. Indication of "alert"/"critical"/"panic" value and whether it has been called to the requesting unit or floor.

Combining manual validation/supplementation with analyzer results

In the concept we have been following, the analytical process consists of all analyses performed on each specimen, both automated and manual. The overall results then consist of information derived from both automated and manual analyses, some of which is overlapping, some of which is complementary and some of which is contradictory. The challenge is to provide a comprehensive report which contains all the useful information which has been derived from automated and manual analyses, but which is not confusing. There are no hard and fast rules. The content of the report for, say, a CBC with differential, will vary, depending on the analyzer's handling of the individual sample, the preferences of the laboratory director and the preferences of the requesting physician.

There are certain general questions which need to be addressed by each specific laboratory:

1. a. If a manual differential is done for any reason, should absolute results from the manual differential and WBC be calculated and reported?
    b. If bands are counted, how should they be reported? For example, should the analyzer total neutrophil count remain and should bands be included in the total neutrophil count?
    c. Should the automated differential be totally or partially replaced with the manual differential?
2. Blood film red cell size estimates: should the analyzer flags for RBC morphology be replaced by the manual estimates? Should an abnormal RDW value remain if blood film review does not confirm anisocytosis?

QUALITY CONTROL STRATEGIES

The first essential for quality control is that there be adequate methods for calibration of the analyzer. These may consist of reference methods, reference materials or calibrators.

CALIBRATION AND STABILITY OF CALIBRATION

Hemoglobin

There are reference procedures for hemoglobin (see Chapter 4). Hemoglobin measurements can be calibrated accurately by spectrophotometric methods. There is also a stable International Standard based on absorptivity of hemiglobin cyanide to which other stable hemoglobin preparations can be referenced—the concept of "traceability".

Hematocrit (PCV)

There are reference procedures for the hematocrit, whereby the hematocrit measurement on a multiparameter analyzer can be referenced to that of the spun hematocrit of fresh whole blood (see Chapter 4). However, as the primary measurement for the analyzers is MCV, it is necessary to have an accurate method for red cell counting

Cell counting

Multiparameter analyzers do not measure absolute quantities of blood and diluent, so it is necessary to calibrate red cell, white cell and platelet counting channels by adjustment to obtain the correct reading on a calibrator preparation. There is no international stable reference material to which red cell, white cell or platelet counts can be referenced. The reference procedure for counting red and white blood cells consists of electronic counting by a single channel, manometer driven cell counter, embodied in the Coulter ZBI®. (See Chapter 4.)

Calibration can be achieved by using these reference methods with several samples of fresh whole blood under rigorous procedures. However, more commonly, a manufacturer of calibration material will assign values to a calibration material by an "indirect" procedure (Groner, 1982) using fresh whole blood on analyzers of the relevant make and model. In the indirect procedure, the analyzer is calibrated with the newly prepared calibration material and results obtained on several fresh human blood samples are compared with results obtained on those same samples by the reference methods. The label values of the calibration material are adjusted until the results on the fresh human blood samples closely match those obtained by the reference methods. This iterative procedure is tedious and time consuming, but must be completed within a few hours of drawing the fresh human blood samples. These commercially produced calibration materials have a stability of 30 to 90 days, depending on the materials used in the preparation.

The WBC differential count

This cannot be calibrated in the usual sense. The integrity of the aperture or flowcell can be set and adjusted; gains can be set; sensitivity can be set; and thresholds can be set to allow the the discriminator or clustering algorithms to function optimally. However, the design of these systems does not allow the user to make adjustments based on reference preparation values to calibrate the differential count.

Internal (intralaboratory) quality control

Quality control is a means to assure the integrity of the analytical process, that is, to detect analytical error. It is part of the larger process of quality assurance, which consists of procedures, including accurate specimen identification, to assure the quality of the entire laboratory operation. Overall quality assurance is beyond the scope of this book. In establishing quality control procedures it is necessary to control for accuracy as well as drift and increased imprecision. Drift refers to a progressive shift of values in one direction, whereas increased imprecision manifests as increased scatter of results from the target value over a period of time. In other words, quality control methods and rules for taking action based on quality control results should detect systematic error (a drift in one direction away from the calibrated set-point) as well as random error (increased imprecision). In deciding what quality control procedures and action rules to use, the aim is to increase the probability of detecting analytical error, while reducing the probability of false rejection of an analytical run.

It is highly desirable that the material used for quality control be as similar as possible in all respects to fresh whole blood, i.e. to patient specimens and that it be subjected to the same procedures as patient specimens, both pre-analytically and analytically. When an analyzer has been calibrated, it is necessary to check that calibration has been achieved successfully, i.e. for accuracy. This is usually achieved by running control samples with known values. Subsequently, it is necessary to check regularly and frequently (at least once per shift) that calibration is being maintained within set tolerance limits, i.e. that drift has not occurred and that imprecision has not increased beyond expected tolerance limits.

Most of the problems related to quality control of hematology analyzers are due to lack of stability. The hydraulic and mechanical components of analyzers are far less stable than the electronic circuits. Lack of stability of control materials is a major problem and is one of the major reasons why several different approaches to many aspects of quality control are used. Many laboratories use a combination of some or all of the approaches discussed below; each has advantages and disadvantages and none is ideal for all aspects of quality control.

Methods for internal quality control

Analysis of preserved commercial material

This is currently the most commonly used approach. Blood cells are stabilized to last for 30 to 45 days. The material has to be optimized for the technology of each analyzer; seldom can such material be used satisfactorily for two analyzers using different technology. Some manufacturers have been able to produce material with a shelf life of 90 days for certain analyzers. Even the 90 day stability is very short when compared with the stability of one to two years of lyophilized and liquid frozen controls for chemistry and coagulation assays. The major difficulty is the preservation of leukocyte types sufficiently well to enable the differential counting algorithms of the analyzer to differentiate them adequately. Manufacturing processes and the constituents of the material are proprietary to each manufacturer and are not disclosed to customers. The blood cells used are mainly human, but porcine, avian and other cells may be used as surrogates. For example, fixed avian red cells, which contain a nucleus, are sometimes used as surrogate white cells.

Values and ranges are assigned to the batch of material at the time of manufacture. The prepared material is analyzed repeatedly on analyzers for which it is designed and a mean value and statistical range of deviation is established.

Stabilized preparations have several disadvantages (Bull, 1991):

1. The material may be inadequately stabilized, so that the cells deteriorate or change their characteristics before the expiration date. If not recognized by the user as failure of the control material itself, time-consuming, expensive troubleshooting, maintenance and recalibration of an analyzer may be undertaken.
2. The material may be overstabilized, usually by excessive fixation, so that the cells behave unlike fresh human cells in the analyzer. For example, overfixation of red cells could reduce deformability; causing errors in size measurement; and could cause resistance to lysis in the white cell channel, causing a falsely high WBC count on the control sample, with interference with the WBC differential count.
3. The cost is high, because of the need for production and rapid shipment of fairly frequent, relatively small batches of control material, with attendant high unit cost of value assignment of the control material by the manufacturer.

Re-analysis of retained patient samples

Patient specimens on which results were obtained when the system was known to be in control are analysed repeatedly through the day. Many laboratories use this for within-day control; some extend it to control the first results of the following day, i.e to 24 hours. The advantage is that this is fresh whole blood; the disadvantage is the lack of stability of the blood regardless of storage conditions. Hemoglobin is stable throughout the day and for 24 hours. Red cell counts will remain stable for 24 hours, especially if the control samples are kept refrigerated; MCV, however, increases. Platelets and leukocytes will deteriorate over 24 hours and changes in values within 24 hours are likely. Depending on the technology of the analyzer, differential counts may remain sufficiently stable for several hours during the day, but may not be stable for 24 hours and are generally adversely affected by cold storage. For a busy laboratory which analyses many specimens throughout the 24 hours, it is feasible to choose different patient specimens for retention at the beginning of each 8 hour shift and re-analyze these throughout that shift.

This method controls for drift and imprecision, but not for accuracy per se.

Moving averages

This approach is based on the notion that the mean value of batches of patient results for an analyte will remain fairly constant over time. This notion appears to be valid for many analytes when only normal patient results are included (Hoffman and Ward, 1965) and holds true for red cell indices (Bull *et al.*, 1974), even when abnormal results are included, provided that the abnormalities are random. Deviations from the mean value are assumed to be due to analytical error. This approach detects systematic error in the most recent batch by comparing its mean value for patient results to the known, previously established patient mean for the analyte.

There are several considerations in the use of this approach:

1. The biological variability of the analyte, compared with the analytic variability. If both are expressed as standard deviation or coefficient of variation, a ratio of biological to analytic variability (S_b/S_a) can be established. The smaller the ratio, the smaller the batch size needed to detect systematic errors. It has been calculated that this ratio is only 1.7 for MCHC (for impedance cell counters), requiring a batch size of 20 to detect an analytical shift of 2 SD with 50% probability. The ratio is 6 for platelets, with required batch size of 70; 7 for MCH, with batch size of 100; 11 for MCV, with batch size of 250; 12 for WBC with a batch size of 300, 16 for hematocrit and RBC with batch size of 400, and 23 for hemoglobin with batch size of 800 (Cembrowski and Carey, 1989). The practicality of this approach depends upon the relationship between the batch size and the

number of samples which are processed during the laboratory turn-around time. If the batch size is smaller than the number of samples then results can be verified before release.

2. The truncation limits for exclusion of patient data. Bull and Korpman (1982) recommended an algorithm which smooths and trims the raw data, minimizing the effect of values far away from the mean. This is now commonly known as "Bull's algorithm" and is programmed into most multiparameter hematology analyzers.

3. The action rules to minimize false rejection of a batch. In a similar manner to results from the analysis of quality control materials, results of each patient batch mean can be compared to the overall mean, and limits of variability can be established. Action rules have to be established to detect analytical errors without excessive false rejection of batches.

4. Initial verification that erythrocyte indices of the patient population are similar to erythrocyte indices elsewhere. It is necessary to establish stable patient mean indices by initially collecting at least 500 consecutive patient values for MCV, MCH and MCHC while maintaining the analyzer in control with commercial preserved control material, over a period of a month. The means are obtained by simple averaging, without using Bull's smoothing and trimming algorithm. Once patient means have been established, batches of 20 samples with application of Bull's algorithm are used to maintain control.

This approach has had most applicability to red cell measurements, especially MCHC, MCH and MCV, and most of all to MCHC. It is useful for detecting systematic error, i.e. drift. Because of the large number of patient samples per batch that would be required, this approach is not useful for leukocytes and platelets.

Action rules

Whichever of the three approaches, singly or in combination, described above is chosen, most modern multiparameter analyzers have the software to accumulate results, display and print them and produce graphs. However, for each of these approaches, rules for taking action have to be established. For example, should any control value which is greater than 2 SD from the mean result in recalibration of the analyzer? This has been extensively studied by using power function curves to model the error detection rate and false rejection rate of various rules. The most widely used rules are some combination of those developed by Westgard (Westgard *et al.*, 1981), initially for chemistry analysis. A subset of these have been applied to hematology (Bull 1991 and Cembrowski, 1989); these are applicable to the quality control approaches described above.

Preserved (commercial) samples:

1. The first consideration is that the manufacturer's expected ranges listed in the package insert of commercially supplied controls generally consider variation among instruments and hence are usually too broad for effective quality control in an individual laboratory. The expected standard deviations for the analyzer in use should be established after installation of the instrument; this will most likely have been done to verify that performance of the analyzer matches the manufacturer's claims for imprecision. Action limits are then applied using this standard deviation.
2. Three different control levels, low, medium and high, are usually analyzed at least once per day and for busy laboratories, at least once per shift. A combination of rules is applicable to these control values.

For the directly measured values (Hb, RBC and MCV): If all control values are within 2 SD of the mean, the analysis is assumed to be in control. If any control result is more than 3 SD from the mean (1_{3s} rule), the analysis is assumed to be out of control and corrective action is taken. If 2 of 3 control results are more than 2 SD from the mean, either on the same side of the mean (the $(2 \text{ of } 3)_{2s}$ rule), or on opposite sides (R_{4s} rule), corrective action is taken. If only the first control value exceeds 2 SD, then the last value from the preceding control run is examined; if this is also greater than 2 SD on the same side of the mean (2_{2s} rule), then corrective action is taken. The consecutive application of these rules is shown in Figure 6.6.

For the calculated results, such as MCH, MCHC and hematocrit, the 1_{3s} rule is adequate, so long as the measured values are controlled by the multi-rule approach described above.

Retained patient samples: Cembrowski *et al.* (1988) studied the effectiveness of various control procedures using retained patient specimens. They found that the variation of red cell measurements (Hb, RBC, MCV, MCH, MCHC and hematocrit) of patient specimens retained and analyzed over a 40 hour period on a Coulter S+IV was equivalent to the variation of a Coulter commercial control product analyzed over 30 days. There was greater variation in the WBC and platelet measurements. Thus control limits for retained specimens can be derived from the long-term standard deviation of commercial controls, with some broadening of the WBC and platelet limits.

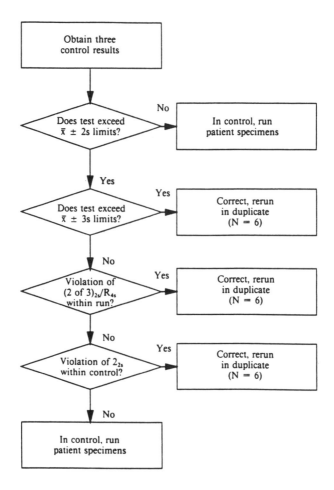

Figure 6.6   Implementation of the $1_{3s}(2$ of $3)_{2s}/R_{4s}$ control procedure. From Cembrowski and Carey (1989) with permission

Cembrowski and co-workers (Cembrowski *et al.*, 1988) suggest that three normal range patient specimens be retained and re-analyzed at regular intervals, for example 8 hourly. In a later paper, Hackney and Cembrowski (1990) modified their suggested program to allow smaller laboratories to use only one retained patient specimen. However, we caution users of the retained specimen approach that they should aerate the retained samples before analysis on each occasion, as MCV rises under anaerobic conditions. Cembrowski *et al.* state that the (2 of 3)$_{2s}$ rule is the most effective rule based on power function analysis and recommend that this be applied only to the directly measured values, i.e. Hb, RBC, MCV, platelets and WBC. The rule will apply when 2 of the 3 retained patient specimens exceeds the difference. Note that the differences here are between the current result and the original result, not between the current result and the mean, as for preserved control material. This method is more sensitive to systematic than to random error.

There is little documentation of the applicability of this approach to the WBC differential. Because of the lack of stability on many analyzers of individual white cell types in patient specimens retained for long periods, this method is probably only applicable within one day and should be used with caution for control for the next day, i.e. the full 24 hour period.

Moving averages: Two rules are usually applied: a test is considered to be out of control either if the Bull average for a batch is greater than 3% different from its usual value in either direction (Bull *et al.*, 1974), or if the average of the last three Bull means is greater than 2% from the usual mean in either direction (Levy *et al.*, 1986). The latter rule is preferable, as it is more sensitive to error for shifts in hemoglobin and MCV, whereas both rules are satisfactory for shifts in RBC count (Lunetzky and Cembrowski, 1987).

Application of quality control methods

Red cell measurements

Preserved control materials, retained patient specimens and moving averages each have utility for these measurements. Each of them can detect systematic error. Random error is best detected by preserved control materials. It is suggested that the most efficient and economical use of these methods is to use three levels of preserved control material at the beginning of each day or each shift and then monitor the remainder of the shift with retained patient specimens and moving averages.

White cell count

Preserved control material and retained patient specimens are useful. Moving averages are not useful for quality control due to the large degree of biologic variability of the WBC. It is suggested that three levels of preserved control material be used at the beginning of each day or each shift, with continuing re-analysis of retained patient samples for ongoing monitoring.

Platelet count

The situation is very similar to that for the WBC. A combination of preserved control material at the beginning of each day or each shift with ongoing re-analysis of retained patient samples should provide satisfactory control. However, platelet counts in retained samples may be found to drop towards the end of the 24 hour period.

WBC dierential count

Counting: The automated WBC differential count is the most problematic for quality control. Manufacturers have experienced difficulty in providing preserved material for WBC differential quality control, particularly for cell types present in low proportions, but reasonably satisfactory material is now available for each specific technology. Retained patient specimens have limited stability for many analyzers. Moving averages are not suitable for quality control of the differential count, due to the wide biologic variability. The manual differential count cannot be used as a quality control check on the analyzer differential count, because of the greater imprecision of the manual count.

The use of three levels of preserved control material designed specifically for the analyzer, at the beginning of each shift, followed by re-analysis of retained patient samples within the time-frame in which the differential count results are stable, provides the most appropriate quality control presently available.

Flagging for abnormals: A further difficult aspect of quality control for the automated WBC differential count is flagging for abnormal cells. Hematologic review of automated analyzer results was discussed above. However, for quality control, the problem is the ability to determine whether flagging characteristics of the analyzer have changed from the time of installation of the analyzer. This question appears to have been largely overlooked, perhaps because there is no direct means for adjustments to be made in the laboratory. In routine operation of the analyzer, false negative flags will not be detected unless some other abnormality causes review of a blood film from the specimen, or a subsequent specimen results in review of a blood film from the first false negatively flagged specimen. A progressive increase in the number of false positive flags will most likely raise concerns eventually, but this is more intuitive than scientific. We are not aware of anyone who has applied any quality control methods to monitor the ongoing performance of hematology analyzers for flagging abnormal cells.

The false positive side of the problem could be addressed by monitoring, perhaps on a daily basis, the percentage of false positive flags produced by the analyzer. To be reasonably certain that the flags are truly false positive, a second, more expert morphologist should also review every slide on which the first observer finds no explanation for the analyzer flag (Bull, 1991). Because of the variability of the proportion of abnormal specimens received by a laboratory from day to day, this approach is fraught with uncertainty and the statistical power of this approach to detect change is obviously low.

Presently, the best approach appears to be that of *quality assurance*. Firstly, this involves strict compliance with regular maintenance procedures at the intervals recommended by the manufacturer for each procedure, especially cleaning; meticulous monitoring of temperatures, voltage levels, hydraulic and vacuum pressures, detector output levels etc. of the analyzer; careful adjustment of gains (amplification), pressures etc. to maintain the analyzer to its specifications; and any other analyzer-specific procedures. Secondly, for false negatives, an explanation should be sought for every significant false negative discovered, including review of previous results and slides where available; there should be discussions with technical representatives of the manufacturer for recurring similar problems, with field service engineer adjustment and repair if necessary. Thirdly, for excessive false positives, keeping a record of each one may enable the laboratory to modify its hematologic review criteria as described above; field service adjustments may also assist if false positive rates have increased greatly. Fourthly, for patients who are admitted to a hospital, many laboratories will perform a blood film review on admission, whether the analyzer hematologic review criteria are triggered or not.

EXTERNAL (INTERLABORATORY) QUALITY CONTROL

External quality control, known also as interlaboratory surveys, or external proficiency surveys, originated in 1946, when Belk and Sunderman sent samples from the same serum pool to 59 laboratories to compare results for several chemistry analytes (Belk and Sunderman, 1947). The College of American Pathologists (CAP) began voluntary chemistry surveys a year later. Since that time, numerous voluntary external quality control surveys have been instituted by professional and national organizations such as UKNEQAS including several for hematology. These programs emphasized self analysis and self improvement by the participants. One of the major goals of the earlier surveys was to diminish interlaboratory variability (Eilers, 1970). There is little doubt that interlaboratory surveys have resulted in improved performance of laboratory testing and have diminished variability between laboratories in all disciplines for which they have been used.

In recent years, regulatory agencies in the United States and elsewhere have adopted interlaboratory surveys for proficiency testing. Satisfactory performance on surveys has become an integral part of required compliance for licensure and accreditation of laboratories. Thus, in some countries the voluntary motive of quality improvement has been replaced by a mandated regulatory requirement for participation.

Although the educational aspects have diminished in several programs as regulatory requirements have increased, some programs, such as those of CAP, maintain a strong educational component, while being deemed acceptable for regulatory purposes by the Federal Government and most States in the US.

Interlaboratory surveys provide a useful form of external quality control for the user of multiparameter hematology analyzers. They enable the laboratory to compare results with other laboratories using the same or similar analyzers on the same samples. This improves uniformity of results among laboratories and may assist in identifying and correcting causes of results which differ greatly from those of other laboratories using the same instruments. Interlaboratory surveys provide information mainly about bias from the mean of the group. However, the duplicate analysis of proficiency samples and other practices (Cembrowski and Vanderlinde, 1988) suggest that interlaboratory surveys used at that time for regulatory purposes probably represented best laboratory performance rather than usual laboratory performance. Most programs for regulatory purposes now require the analyst as well as the laboratory director to sign attestation statements that the proficiency samples were handled and tested identically (as far as practicable) to patient specimens.

There are several cautions in the use of external surveys and interpretation of results for quality control purposes:

1. As for all quality control specimens, the ideal sample should be as similar to fresh human blood as possible. This is rarely possible, except for small studies within a geographically confined area. The survey samples need to be stable for at least a few weeks to allow for manufacture, dispensing, shipment and analysis by participating laboratories. Thus, samples are preserved in some fashion and may not be analysed adequately in all respects.

2. Because of the different technologies in different analyzers, the material may not perform equally well on all analyzers. This is particularly noticeable for the differential count; CAP now provides different samples to laboratories using analyzers with different technology, each sample being optimized in its manufacture for each technology.

3. Comparison of analyzer results with those of other analyzers using the same reagent systems is necessary, because of the different technologies and differences which occur even between models from the same manufacturer.

4. Different methods for calibration and use of different calibrators for the same make and model of analyzer may cause greater variability within that group, compared with a group where the same calibrator is used.

5. The group of participants providing results for a particular analyzer may be too small to provide statistically valid results. The small group may then be included in a larger group which may be inappropriate because of technology differences. More subtle is the fact that larger groups tend to have smaller standard deviations; this may be a function of group size, or merely that there is more likely to be a number of laboratories using very similar calibration material and procedures. Thus the standard deviation within a smaller group may appear much greater. Results of interlaboratory surveys should be used with great caution in comparisons of instrument quality.

6. Because of the unavoidable delay in returning results to the participating laboratories and the infrequency of most surveys, these results have little impact on the day-to-day operation of the analyzers and the laboratory. They do help to provide assurance of uniformity among laboratories and can help to identify persistent trends in an individual laboratory.

In addition to interlaboratory surveys provided by certain States, such as New York State and those offered by professional organizations such as CAP and NEQAS, manufacturers of some instruments and quality control materials now provide interlaboratory programs as part of their service to customers. Many of these manufacturer programs include the daily quality control results in their analysis, thus providing the laboratory with information concerning its within-day drift and imprecision as compared with other users, as well as overall bias between the laboratory and the consensus mean of the same model instrument in other laboratories.

As more hematology laboratories seek higher levels of laboratory automation, the need for integration of multiparameter analyzers into hematology laboratories becomes more widespread. Manufacturers are responding by increasing the features of their systems and improving the user-interface with their systems, as well as developing new approaches to laboratory automation. The direction of future developments is rather clear in many respects, and will be discussed in some detail in the next chapter.

REFERENCES

Banez, E.L. and Bacaling, H.D. (1988) An evaluation of the Technicon H*1 automated hematology analyzer in detecting peripheral blood changes in acute inflammation. *Arch. Pathol. Lab. Med.* **112**: 885–8.

Baron, M.A. and Fink, H.D. (1980) Bacteremia in private pediatric practice. *Pediatrics* **66**: 171–5.

Belk, W.P. and Sunderman, F.W. (1947) A survey of the accuracy of chemical analysis in clinical laboratories. *Am. J. Clin. Pathol.* **17**: 853–61.

Brigden, M.L. and Page, N.E. (1990) The lack of clinical utility of white blood cell differential counts and blood morphology in elderly individuals with normal hematology profiles. *Arch. Pathol. Lab. Med.* **114**: 394–8.

Bull, B.S. (1991) Quality assurance strategies. In Koepke, J. (ed.) *Laboratory Hematology*, 2nd edn, pp. 3–29. Churchill–Livingstone, London.

Bull, B.S. and Korpman, R.A. (1982) Intra-laboratory quality control using patients' data. In Cavill, I. (ed.) *Methods in Hematology*, Vol. 4. pp. 121–150. *Quality Control*. Churchill-Livingstone, New York.

Bull, B.S., Elashoff, R.M., Heilbron, A.C. and Couperus. J. (1974) A study of various estimators for the derivation of quality control procedures from patient erythrocyte indices. *Am. J. Clin. Pathol.* **61**: 473–81.

Cembrowski, G.S. and Carey, A.R. (1989) Quality control in hematology. In Cembrowski, G.S. and Carey, A.R. (eds.) *Laboratory Quality Management*. American Society of Clinical Pathology, Chicago, IL.

Cembrowski, G.S. and Carey, A.R. (1989) *Laboratory Management QC/QA*. pp. 197–8. American Society of Clinical Pathology, Chicago, IL.

Cembrowski, G.S. and Vanderlinde, R. (1988) Survey of special practices associated with College of American Pathologists proficiency testing in the Commonwealth of Pennsylvania. *Arch. Pathol. Lab. Med.* **112**: 374–6.

Cembrowski, G.S., Lunetzky, E.S., Patrick, C.C. and Wilson, M.K. (1988) Optimized quality control procedure for hematology analyzers using retained patient specimens. *Am. J. Clin. Pathol.* **89**: 203–10.

Christensen, R.D., Bradley, P.P. and Rothstein, G. (1981) The leucocyte left shift in clinical and experimental neonatal sepsis. *J. Pediatr.* **98**: 101–5.

Dueholm, S., Bagi, P. and Bud, M. (1989) Laboratory aid in the diagnosis of acute appendicitis: a blinded prospective trial concerning diagnostic value of leukocyte count, neutrophil differential count and C-reactive protein. *Dis. Colon Rectum* **32**: 855–9.

Dutcher, T.F. (1984) Leukocyte differentials. Are they worth the effort? *Clin. Lab. Med.* **4**: 71–87.

Eilers, R.J. (1970) Total quality control for the medical laboratory: the role of the College of American Pathologists Survey Program. *Am. J. Clin. Pathol.* **54**: 435–6.

Groner, W. (1982) Standardization of multi-parameter instruments for blood cell blood cell counting and sizing. In Cavill, I. (ed.) *Methods in Hematology: Quality Control*, 2nd Edn, pp. 13–34. Churchill–Livingstone, London.

Hackney, J.R. and Cembrowski, G.S. (1990) The use of retained patient specimens for haematology quality control. *Clin. Lab. Haematol.* **12**: (Suppl 1): 83–89.

Hayashi, M. (1992) The Sysmex Total Hematology System. *Sysmex J. Int.* **2**: 96–102.

Hoffman, R.G. and Waid, N.E. (1965) The "average of normals" method of quality control. *Am. J. Clin. Pathol.* **43**: 134–41.

Levy, W.C., Hay, K.L. and Bull, B.S. (1986) Preserved blood versus patient data for quality control—Bull's algorithm revisited. *Am. J. Clin. Pathol.* **85**: 719–21.

Lotspeich-Steininger, C.A., Stiene-Martin, E.A. and Koepke, J.A. (1992) *Clinical Hematology: Principles, Procedures, Correlations*, pp. 10–19. Lippincott, Philadelphia, New York.

Lunetzky, E.S. and Cembrowski, G.S. (1985) Performance characteristics of Bull's multi-rule algorithm for the quality control of multichannel hematology analyzers. *Am. J. Clin. Pathol.* **83**: 337–45.

Marchand, A., van Lente, F. and Galen, R.S. (1983) The assessment of laboratory tests in the diagnosis of acute appendicitis. *Am. J. Clin. Pathol.* **80**: 369–74.

NCCLS (1991a) *Protection of Laboratory Workers from Infectious Disease Transmitted by Blood, Body Fluids, and Tissue*, 2nd Edn. Tentative Guideline NCCLS Document M29-T2, NCCLS, Villanova, PA.

NCCLS (1991b) *Procedures for the Collection of Diagnostic Blood Specimens by Venipuncture*, 3rd Edn. Approved Standard. NCCLS Document H3-A3. NCCLS, Villanova PA.

NCCLS (1992) *Reference Leukocyte Differential Count (Proportional) and Evaluation of Instrumental Methods; Approved Standard*. NCCLS Document H20-A. NCCLS, Villanova, PA.

NCCLS (1993a) *Methods for the Erythrocyte Sedimentation Rate (ESR) Test*, 3rd Edn. Approved Standard, NCCLS Document H2-A3. NCCLS, Villanova, PA.

NCCLS (1993b) *Procedure for Determining Packed Cell Volume by the Microhematocrit Method*, 2nd Edn. Approved Standard, NCCLS Document H7-A2. NCCLS, Villanova, PA.

Todd, J.K. (1974) Childhood infections. Diagnostic value of peripheral white blood cell and differential cell counts. *Am. J. Dis. Child* **127**: 810–16.

Wasserman, M., Levinstein, M., Keller, E., Lee, S. and Yoshikawa, T.T. (1989) Utility of fever, white blood cells, and differential count in predicting bacterial infections in the elderly. *J. Amer. Geriat. Soc.* **37**: 537–43.

Wenz, B., Ramirez, M.A. and Burns, E.R. (1987) The H*1 hematology analyzer. Its performance characteristics and value in the diagnosis of infectious disease. *Arch. Pathol. Lab. Med.* **111**: 521–4.

Westgard, J.O., Barry, P.L., Hunt, M.R. and Groth, T. (1981) A multirule Shewhart chart for quality control in clinical chemistry. *Clin. Chem.* **27**: 493–501.

Chapter 7

Future Developments

INTRODUCTION

The fundamental purpose of the current cell counting instrument systems described in the previous chapters is the automation of diagnostic procedures of long standing in routine hematology, namely, the examination of the peripheral blood film. A great deal of progress toward this goal has been made in the past decade. A number of systems are now available which automatically analyze fresh blood and produce 20 or more parameters measuring properties of the blood cells. In most cases, these provide a reasonable and complete diagnostic picture equivalent in quality and superior in precision to the microscopic review of the blood film by a competent morphologist. However, it has also been shown that substantial remaining issues limit both the easy integration of the modern systems into the routine hematology laboratory and the full medical benefits of the results. Notably:

1. The automated analysis is not complete and requires manual follow-up in a substantial fraction of the specimens encountered in the typical routine hematology laboratory.
2. The diagnostic value of the results in abnormal blood specimens is still limited since the current systems merely flag specimens and do not report or discriminate among abnormal cells.
3. The results obtained with different systems, especially with regard to the automated leukocyte differential, size parameters and flags, are not standardized. Therefore, the potential clinical value of the increased precision and new parameters is not fully realized.

It was also pointed out in the first chapter that, while the current phase of consolidation and automation of current diagnostic testing was proceeding in the routine laboratory, a period of discovery was flourish-

Practical Guide to Modern Hematology Analyzers. W. Groner and E. Simson
© 1995 John Wiley & Sons Ltd

ing in research laboratories driven by the isolation of key cytokines and the exploitation of more specific labels (monoclonal antibodies and DNA probes) for tagging blood cells and exploring their function.

This chapter will explore the potential for further developments and improvements in routine hematology testing. In performing this review attention will be paid to three areas:

- First we will discuss incremental improvements in the current systems, which in the near term could improve their utility by directly addressing the outstanding issues which were listed above, relying on technology which is currently available.
- Second we will consider some applications of developing technology such as robotics and computer science which may further the trend in automation of the routine hematology laboratory by (more originally) addressing the issues of specimen handling and data processing in more innovative ways.
- Finally we will consider the trends in clinical research and the impact of these trends on the activities in the hematology laboratory of the future.

NEAR-TERM IMPROVEMENTS IN MULTIPARAMETER CELL COUNTERS

The discussion in the previous two chapters has detailed the complications in using modern cell counting systems, which arise from their inability to process all of the specimens automatically. In addition, it has been shown how a great deal of the potential for improvement in the clinical value of reported results which might have been anticipated (as a result of the greater precision in cell counting as well as the new parameters describing cell size) is not realized in practice because of the lack of standardization.

Although great progress has been made, the microscope has not been eliminated in the routine hematology laboratory since visual microscopy is still required on a substantial number of the specimens. Visual microscopy remains as a workstation with complicated logistics since the specimens which require microscopic review are not identified upon accession but rather after testing on the multiparameter cell counter. Thus, the output of the laboratory still consists of a mixture of results obtained from automated cell counters and microscopic analysis. However, in the laboratory which uses modern cell counting systems the mixture is now specimen dependent as opposed to test dependent. That is, a neutrophil percentage obtained on one specimen may be derived from an automated cell counter while the same reported parameter on another specimen may have been derived from a microscopic differential.

It is not likely that these issues will be resolved in the short term since their resolution will probably require the introduction of new technology in instrument systems for the hematology laboratory. However, it is reasonable to anticipate incremental improvements in the equipment and materials available to the hematology laboratory which utilize current available technology to minimize the impact of these issues on laboratory workflow. In particular, one can envision a greater use of robotics, computer science, artificial intelligence (expert systems), and flow cytometry as well as the development of practice standards as short-term improvements in modern cell counters.

ROBOTICS IN THE HEMATOLOGY LABORATORY

Laboratories can generally be described in terms of the number of workstations. Specimen and material flow between the workstations is generally accomplished by manual means. Data flow between workstations is generally accomplished by a combination of manual entry and the Laboratory Information System. Studies of laboratory cost have consistently shown (Bull, 1978) that a substantial fraction of the labor costs are expended at the interface between separate stations. This is especially true when the same specimen must be processed at two or more workstations and then the data collated for reporting. This is a typical situation in the routine hematology laboratory where a profile of results is generally requested in the form of a "complete blood count" (CBC).

Much of the improvement in automating the hematology laboratory has resulted from the consolidation of the workstations required to complete the CBC. Starting in the 1960s with the first automated CBC instruments, until the current multiparameter cell counters, the trend has been to eliminate workstations by combining the functions of two or more workstations in a single instrument. There are limitations in this approach, especially when diverse technology is required. In this case consolidation of workstations can lead to large monolithic instruments which are difficult to obtain because of their initial cost and expensive to maintain because of their complexity. An alternative approach to eliminating the interface workload is through the use of conveyance systems and robotics.

In 1992 Sysmex initiated the use of robotics in the hematology laboratory when they introduced a totally automated hematology analysis system. This system integrates the cell counter with computerized data management and automated specimen handling. The system uses a track to move specimens past connected workstations which include (in addition to the multiparameter cell counter) preparation of a blood film, and a reticulocyte counter. The system is capable of selectively processing the specimen with regard to generating a blood film or obtaining a reticulocyte count on the basis of the results from the multiparameter cell counter. That is, only the specimens requiring additional tests are processed. Thus, although the number of specimens requiring follow-up is not reduced, the manual labor input for hematological review is reduced.

This concept of specimen handling with robotics is also being developed by Coulter for the hematology laboratory and by other manufacturers for use in the serum chemistry laboratory. These devices operate in a similar manner, with separate workstations connected to a specimen transport track. However, in most cases selection of the tests is made at specimen accession and downloaded to the analysis systems by means of the Laboratory Information System. It is likely that in the near term this technology will become widely used in large laboratories to improve the performance of modern cell counters by reducing costs for the laboratory. The current systems both in the chemistry and hematology laboratory are generally limited to the equipment of a single manufacturer. This is because the most difficult challenge is providing a common interface for the connected stations. However, proposals have been made for standards in specimen collection, labeling, and transport. If approved these standards could provide a common interface specification and allow the coupling of instruments made by different manufacturers. The laboratory information system could then be exploited to implement protocols for testing such as autoverification, which is discussed in the next section.

AUTOVERIFICATION

Another advance which utilizes computer technology within the state of the art is autoverification. In this approach (which is also being developed for the chemistry laboratory) the process of detecting and verifying aberrant specimen results is relegated to the Laboratory Information System. Verified results are reported without human intervention. Thus, a time consuming, labor intensive and error prone manual process is eliminated.

Data from the measurements on a specimen are added to the information system database and evaluated. They are scrutinized for validity, cause for concern, or the need for further action prior to reporting. The verification of results depends on the laboratory policy regarding result reporting. This may include delta checks, reference ranges, review flags etc. Typical criteria used by the software are illustrated schematically in Figure 7.1. Table 7.1 shows a trial software configura-

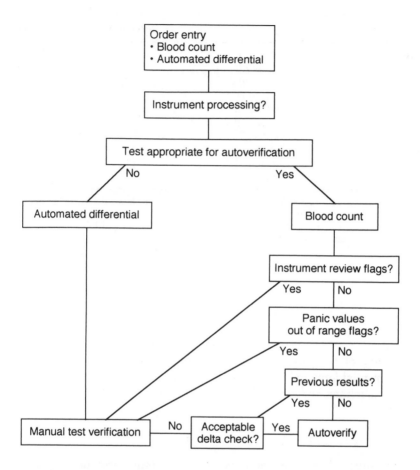

Figure 7.1 Workflow diagram illustrating algorithm used for autoverification. From Davis (1994) with permission

tion for autoverification in hematology (Davis, 1994). Results inconsistent with these criteria are manually verified. The percentage or value controls the amount of deviation from the previous result that is accepted as passing the delta check.

In Table 7.1 the WBC is eligible for verification if the result lies between 2000 and 20 000. If the difference between the current value and the previous value is less than 50% of the previous value the result passes delta check. It is seen that the magnitude of biologic variation (see Chapter 5) has been taken into consideration in formulating the table.

Table 7.1   Autoverification standards of software configuration*

Detail test	Range	Percentage	Value
WBC	2.0 to 20.0	50	NA
RBC	2.0 to 7.0	50	NA
Hb	8.0 to 20.0	NA	4.0
HCT	23.0 to 60.0	NA	12.0
MCV	50.0 to 110.0	NA	3.0
MCH	None	10	NA
MCHC	30.0 to 36.0	NA	3.0
RDW	None	NA	2.5
PLT	30 to 800	50	NA
MPV	None	NA	2.5

*WBC indicates white blood cell; RBC, red blood cell; Hb, hemoglobin; HCT, hematocrit; MCV, mean corpuscular volume; MCH, mean corpuscular hemoglobin; MCHC, mean corpuscular hemoglobin concentration; RDW, red cell distribution width; PLT, platelet count; MPV, mean platelet volume; NA, not applicable.
From Davis (1994) with permission.

The trial configuration illustrated in the table was used in an experiment and the impact on misidentified specimens and specimen turnaround time which was reported is shown in Tables 7.2 and 7.3. The sensitivity of the autoverification configuration with respect to mislabeled or misidentified specimens was 100%. In addition a 57% reduction in specimen turnaround time was noted.

STANDARDIZATION OF CURRENT PRACTICE

One avenue of current activity which should provide improvement in current practice in the near term is to standardize it. Toward this end, collaborative groups of scientists representing both the manufacturers and users of cell counters have been engaged in the development of reference methods and practice standards. As pointed out in Chapter 4 two organizations which are significant in this area are the ICSH and the NCCLS. Recently, these groups have been working on the methods and practice standards in three areas which are worthy of discussion.

1. Methods for calibration and quality control of multiparameter cell counters.
2. Reference methods and standards for the analysis of cell size distribution.
3. Reference methods and evaluation of the leukocyte differential.

Table 7.2 Impact of autoverification on instrument flags and misidentified specimens

	Blood surveys	Autoverification*		Percentage autoverified
		Yes	No	
With instrument flags	41	21	20	50
Without instrument flags	123	76	47	62
Ringers*	23	0	23	0

*Test situation mislabels.
From Davis (1994) with permission.

Table 7.3 Autoverification specimen turnaround time comparison

	Before*	After*	% Reduction
Drawn time to verified time	70.5	59.91	15.02
Time received in lab to verified time	44.6	19.12	57.13

*In minutes.
From Davis (1994) with permission.

Methods for calibrating and quality control of multiparameter cell counters

It was pointed out previously that currently only five reference methods exist for the calibration of modern cell counters when the minimum required is six. In addition, it was demonstrated in Chapter 5 (while reviewing the performance of modern systems) that the current reference method for the white blood cell differential (NCCLS H20-A), which is based on a 400 cell microscope differential, is inadequate for standardizing the automated differential systems as a result of the wide range of variability that is present within the sampling error of 400 cells. Thus, there is considerable development required with regards to creating a menu of reference methods to be used in assigning values to calibrators for the modern cell counting systems and/or evaluating their performance.

The ICSH cytometry panel is addressing the need for reference methods by developing reference methods for the mean cell volume and the indirect platelet count.

Another area in which practice standards could be effective is quality control. The NCCLS sub-committee on quantitative cellular analysis is currently working on a performance standard for the quality control of multiparameter cell counters. This standard will be based upon the relationship between analytical variability and biologic variability as discussed in Chapter 5. It will set performance goals for cell counters and describe methods for verifying performance to these goals.

Reference methods for cell size distribution analysis

The ICSH cytometry panel has also been developing standard practices regarding the analysis of cell size distributions. The first publication General Principles (ICSH, 1982) was published in 1982 and introduced the concept of log normal curve analysis for the size distribution of blood cells. A second publication (ICSH, 1988) further elaborated the curve fitting procedure to be used in obtaining numerical values from a cell size distribution. The panel is now developing reference methods for the size analysis of red blood cells.

Standardizing the white blood cell differential

In parallel with the development of multiparameter cell counters the research and clinical applications of flow cytometry have been growing in the past two decades. The major advances in this field have been in the use of specific monoclonal antibodies together with fluorescent stains to tag a particular class of leukocyte. Principal applications have been for the typing of lymphocytes and classifying leukemia. In each case the exquisite specificity of the monoclonal antibody label has been useful in identification and counting sub-classes of leukocytes. Thus, in a very real sense cells are defined by their reaction to a specific mono-clonal antibody and this definition may be standardized. As an example, consider the CD4+ lymphocyte which is monitored in indivi-duals who are HIV positive. The definition of this helper lymphocyte is made not in terms of morphology but in terms of a cluster density (CD4+) identified by a particular monoclonal antibody. This definition is much more amenable to quality control than a description of cell morphology. Examples from interlaboratory trials (Hamburger *et al.*, 1989) have shown this definition to be standard, and total analytic variability of CD4+ cells as a fraction of leukocytes to be much smaller than that achieved in the leukocyte differential either with the micro-scope or with current multiparameter cell counters. Thus, one means of improving uniformity of automated cell counts could be to define the leukocyte sub-classes in terms of their reaction to specific monoclonal antibodies. Currently, monoclonal antibodies have been demonstrated which label several of the mature sub-classes of leukocytes.

Terstappen (Terstappen *et al.*, 1991) has also reported the use of a combination of monoclonal antibodies with a fluorescent nuclear stain as an alternative means to obtain multiparameter cell counts including a five part WBC differential with multidimensional fluorescent flow cytometry.

ADDITIONAL CELL CLASSIFICATIONS

Another potential for using monoclonal antibodies and flow cytometry in the near term is to extend the classification further than the five mature leukocyte classes. This could allow cell counters to classify and enumerate the cells in abnormal specimens resulting in lower requirements for visual examination of the peripheral blood film.

Thus, the powerful technology of flow cytometry combined with the specific cell tagging afforded by monoclonal antibodies has the potential to address the two remaining issues of automating the leukocyte differential. It may be standardized, and extended to the classification of abnormal specimens. However, fulfilling this potential will require further advances both in flow cytometry and in cell counting. Notably:

1. The monoclonal antibody cell tagging methods used in flow cytometry are generally too long and complex to be considered as part of a multiparameter cell counter.
2. The monoclonal antibody cell tagging methods used in flow cytometry frequently require cell washing or other procedures which lose the account of volume. Thus, they are not suitable for use in cell counters.
3. Monoclonal antibodies are presently directed only to molecules appearing on the surface of the cells and this may not provide sufficient range for identification of abnormal cells.
4. Monoclonal antibodies are expensive and therefore a wide battery of monoclonal antibodies could not be considered practical for use on every specimen in a profile. Cell counters would have to be developed which employed only selective applications of the antibodies.

TECHNOLOGY TRENDS

The previous section discussed improvements to modern multiparameter cell counters which might result from application of technology within the state of the art in the context of integrating modern cell counting systems into the routine hematology laboratory. In this section we will consider trends in technology which are liable to affect the hematology laboratory by creating new products or methods which use technology essentially different from that in current use to address the key open issue of automating the CBC + WBC differential. That is, reducing the need for hematological review by extending the automation to abnormal specimens.

Areas which will be considered include:

1. Re-emergence of image analysis on blood films.
2. Combination of flow cytometer and image analysis
3. Use of fluorescent methods for cell tagging.
4. Automated reflex testing.
5. Automated analysis of abnormal cytograms by computer.

RE-EMERGENCE OF IMAGE ANALYSIS ON BLOOD FILMS

It was pointed out in Chapter 1 that the first attempts to automate the WBC differential were made by direct application of computer pattern recognition analysis to the stained peripheral blood film. Although this method was not successful at that time some of the reasons for failure have been removed by advances in computer technology. Computer speed is much greater today and is becoming quite capable of competing with flow cytometery (Shack *et al.*, 1987; Kamentsky and Kamentsky, 1991). In addition, computer hardware is now less expensive and allows the use of sophisticated algorithms for cell identification including learning algorithms.

Unfortunately, some of the problems with this approach still remain which limit the analysis of the blood film as the basic technology for multiparameter cell counting. The most notable of these is the loss of volume accounting between the blood film and the original specimen. That is, it is not possible to relate directly the cells per unit area on the blood film to the cells per unit volume in the whole blood specimen. This precludes the use of this technology for volume sensitive cell counts such as RBC, WBC, and platelet counts. However, image analysis does provide a more extensive data set on abnormal cells and could provide the means to extend cell counting to more abnormal cell specimens eliminating the need for hematological review. In order to be effective means would have to be provided to couple the image analysis station to the cell counting station. This could be accomplished by coupling the workstations through the use of automated conveyance and robotics as discussed above or, alternatively, by combining a flow cytometer with image analysis as we will discuss below.

COMBINATION OF FLOW CYTOMETER AND IMAGE ANALYSIS.

Recent results have been reported with cell counting systems that combine some of the features of flow cytometers with image analysis.

Two reports are of more than routine interest: the "White IRIS" (Kasdan *et al.*, 1994) and "Volumetric Capillary Cytometry" (Manian *et al.*, 1994).

The White IRIS system, which is developed and marketed by International Remote Imaging Systems, uses a slow sheath stream flow cell and a stop action scan to digitize cell images as they pass through an optical detection station. The system uses 2-methylpolymethine as a supravital stain which induces metachromasia in the leukocytes. Leukocytes are concentrated before analysis by aggregating the red blood cells and then using density fractionation. Thus, volume accounting is lost and only a differential WBC count is achieved. Five hundred WBCs are classified into ten categories which include, in addition to the five mature classes, bands, metamyelocytes, myelocytes, promyelocytes and blast cells. Figure 7.2 shows a photograph of the White IRIS system.

The Volumetric Capillary Cytometry (VCC) approach being developed by Biometric Imaging optically scans a cell suspension while temporarily stopped in a capillary flow cell of precise dimensions. Thus, volume accounting is maintained. However, the current methods being developed for this system are limited to the sub-classes of lymphocytes, which are fluorescently labelled with a monoclonal antibody.

In each of these systems a digitized image of certain blood cells is analyzed by computer. Spatial resolution is not as great as can be achieved with cells spread out on a microscope slide. However, sufficient data may be obtained to extend to the classification of abnormal cells, especially when the technique employs a combination of cell tagging and image analysis, as in the White IRIS system.

USE OF FLUORESCENT METHODS FOR CELL TAGGING

During the same period that the multiparameter cell counters described in this book were developed and integrated into routine hematology laboratories, flow cytometers were being used in research. It was pointed out above that the fundamental difference between a flow cytometer and a cell counter is the issue of volume accounting. Another practical difference was the use of fluorescent tagging methods in research flow cytometers. These methods were suitable for use in the research laboratory but the instruments required high power lasers, and were generally not considered practical for use in the routine laboratory.

Recently advances in lasers and in cell tagging fluorescent dyes have made the use of fluorescent tagging more practical. Laser diodes are now available with substantial power density in the red region of the visible spectrum. Further, several useful dyes that excite in the same region of the spectrum have also been developed. By combining these two technologies it now appears reasonable that the future will see

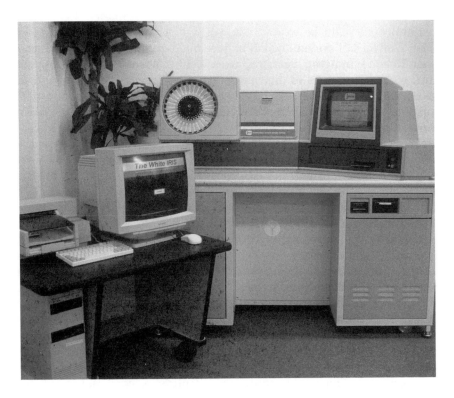

Figure 7.2 Photograph of the "White IRIS" system. Courtesy of International
Remote Imaging Systems, Chatsworth, CA, USA

fluorescent tags in use in cell counters which are no more complex than
the current cell counting instruments which use optical detection technology for cell classification. These instruments will be able to use more
specific tags as a result of the higher sensitivity of fluorescent labeling.
Thus, they may provide a practical platform to combine cell counting
with fluorescent tagging and enable the use of monoclonal antibodies
for recognition and the classification of a larger number of cell categories including abnormal cells.

AUTOMATED REFLEX TESTING

In the section on incremental improvements to current cell counting
systems, application of state of the art technology to the problem of
hematological review for flagged specimens was addressed. Two

approaches were considered; automated conveyance and robotics to interface workstations, and autoverification. In the more distant future these concepts could be extended to fully automate the review process through the use of automated reflex testing. Reflex testing is the performance of a second test based on the results obtained in the first test. That is, initiating a follow-up test to obtain further data on an abnormal specimen. The concept described as autoverification could be extended to proceed with further tests which are only applied to the specimen when the results are not verified.

Sysmex has already begun this process with the selective method of generating a peripheral blood film in their Total Automated Laboratory. In this device blood films are generated at the request of a computer which has been programmed to select only those specimens requiring hematological review for film generation. Results from the NE-8000 cell counter are used to determine which specimens require a blood film and also to adjust the angle and speed of film generation based on the hematocrit, to obtain an optimal blood film. A similar concept could be used to trigger further analysis by image analysis or by selected monoclonal antibodies. In this way the added costs or time for processing abnormal specimens can be limited to only those specimens flagged in the original pass.

One incremental step along this direction is the Micro 21 system developed by Intelligent Medical Imaging Inc. In this system an automated microscope is used to provide a hematological review of abnormal specimens. The microscope automatically classifies WBCs into up to 11 categories including blast cells, nucleated red blood cells, and sub-classification of immature granulocytes, saving these for operator confirmation. Red blood cell morphology is also noted and a platelet estimate is made. Figure 7.3 illustrates the Micro 21 system.

AUTOMATED DIAGNOSIS BY ANALYSIS OF CYTOGRAMS

Another means of eliminating the need for microscopic review of abnormal specimens is to extend the analysis of the cytograms which are obtained with current cell counters on abnormal specimens. The objective would be to replace the need for hematological review by developing a diagnosis based upon the cytograms.

Normal cytograms are very similar to each other, but abnormal cytograms vary quite a lot and have a very large number of different sets of cell distributions. The diagnosis of disease is not only dependent on the cell counts but also on the cell distributions (patterns) of the cytograms. On current multiparameter cell counting systems, extensive flags are used for the abnormal cell populations and conditions. These flags are then used to initiate a hematology review typically performed by a

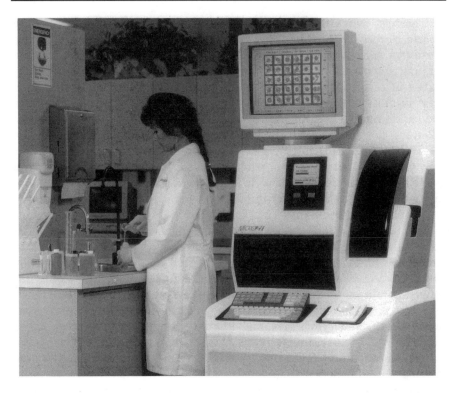

Figure 7.3 Photograph of the Micro 21, fully automated "walk away" micro-scopy. Courtesy of Intelligent Medical Imaging Inc. Palm Beach, FL, USA

microscopic review of the peripheral blood film. One means of eliminat-ing the requirement for hematologic review would be to complete the analysis of the abnormal specimen by a more sophisticated analysis of the cytograms using computer learning. Human analysis and interpre-tation of cytograms to suggest diagnosis has been well developed for certain analyzers (Simson, 1984; Simson *et al.*, 1988). Obviously, the results of such an analysis cannot be equivalent to microscopic review. However, it is conceivable to approach the problem by considering the end result to be an automated diagnosis. The abnormal cytograms consist of valuable clinical information which may assist in directly developing the diagnosis (or alternatively diagnosis probability tables) for various diseases or disorders. This is, of course, not a trivial problem since the information is limited and the number of potential diagnoses quite broad. However, an approach using hierarchical classifi-cation might be combined with either fuzzy sets or neural networks to overcome the difficulty and emulate human thought processes for cyto-gram interpretation.

The algorithms for a hierarchical pattern recognition model for automatic speech recognition (without a teacher) have been outlined by Ornstein (1993) in his paper ("Hierarchic Heuristic: relevance to economic pattern-recognition and high speed data-processing"). As indicated in this paper, the situation appears to be somewhat different in the multidimensional space occupied by human diseases. "Disease Space" does not necessarily contain the large empty gaps between clusters that make "natural" subdivision easy. Although it would not be adequate if an automated diagnosis machine were only able to recognize one out of three or four diseases from which a patient may suffer, a hierarchical taxonomic classification model may be easily extended to deal usefully with fuzzy sets, such as those encountered in medical diagnosis.

The pioneering application of the theory of fuzzy sets to cluster analysis was made in 1969 by Russini. It was not until 1973, however, when the appearance of the work by Dunn and Bezdek on the fuzzy isodata (fuzzy c-means) algorithms became a landmark in the theory of cluster analysis, that the relevance of the theory of fuzzy sets to cluster analysis and pattern recognition became clearly established. Many papers applying the theory of fuzzy sets to medical diagnosis (fuzzy clustering algorithms for cluster validity, fuzzy partitioning algorithm for pattern classification, fuzzy dissimiliture relation for pattern recognition, etc.) have been published.

TRENDS IN CLINICAL RESEARCH AND PRACTICE

The previous sections in this chapter have dealt with the means to improve automation in the current hematology laboratory by extending automated analysis to abnormal specimens or by automating the interface between the cell counter and the microscope. The assumption made was that the test requests were constant. However, medical practice is changing as a result of new discoveries in clinical research. Therefore, it is interesting also to consider a future for the hematology laboratory in which either new tests are ordered or the relative volume of tests changes as a result of changes in the practice of medicine.

In this section we will consider the potential impact on testing in the hematology laboratory resulting from new discoveries or changes in the practice of clinical medicine. Two areas are worthy of discussion:

1. The use of cytokines in therapy.
2. New methods of specific cell recognition through the use of nucleic probes with in-situ hybridization.

THE USE OF CYTOKINES IN THERAPY

Recent years have brought about the isolation cloning, and therapeutic use of specific agents (called cytokines) which stimulate the growth of a target cell line. The most dramatic example is erythropoietin (EPO) which has been successfully used in the treatment of anemia associated with red cell production deficiency. EPO has now also been widely tried with the anemia associated with cancer. Other cytokines have been isolated and cloned for stimulating neutrophils, lymphocytes and platelets. Thus, it is reasonable to assume a more widespread use of cytokine therapy in the future.

This change in therapeutic strategy will impact testing in the hematology laboratory as clinicians attempt to verify the course of the therapy. The attention will be on those tests which measure either more rapidly or more precisely the cell turnover. For instance, the use of EPO will stimulate the counting of reticulocytes as a means to rapidly assess the new red blood cells. Therefore, with the wider use of this drug one can expect an increase in requests for reticulocyte counts.

Recent reports have focused on the discovery of a material which acts to stimulate production of platelets (Metcalf, 1994). In analogy to the use of EPO it is likely that this drug will be used to correct thrombocytopenia which results from lack of production. One obvious application is in combination with cytotoxic therapy used to treat leukemia and other cancers. In this situation the dosage is frequently constrained due to the dangers of lowering the platelet count. Combining with an agent which stimulates platelet production would eliminate this concern. Requests for accurate platelet counts and/or reticulated platelet percentage in thrombocytopenic specimens may increase dramatically to follow therapy with "Thrombopoietin".

Treatment regimens involving drugs which stimulate production of specific leukocyte sub-classes are also being investigated and it is likely that these studies will also provoke requests for precisely counting the number of cells within a certain class to follow the changes induced by the therapy.

In summary, the result of the wider use of cytokines may cause a major shift in the hematology laboratory as test requests become more specific. Thus, the current view of routine hematology as a profiling laboratory with most of the activity focused on the complete blood count may, in the future, give way to a routine hematology laboratory with much more selective testing. A similar trend was seen in the serum chemistry laboratory when profiling was replaced by more selective test protocols. The result in that case was a dramatic change in the type of instruments used in the laboratory. In analogy one may look forward to a similar change in cell counting instruments. The focus of the cell counters of the future might be to automate random selective testing on specimens. These cell counters may perform from 1 to 10 specific cell counts on each specimen by choosing from a wide selection of specific cell tagging methods including monoclonal antibodies and DNA probes which are hybridized within the target.

NEW METHODS OF SPECIFIC CELL RECOGNITION THROUGH THE USE OF NUCLEIC PROBES WITH IN-SITU HYBRIDIZATION

Recent research reports have demonstrated the ability to locate a specific nucleic acid sequence, replicate it, and tag the cell containing the sequence with a fluorescent dye. This technology known as fluorescent in-situ hybridization (FISH) allows exquisite specificity to be applied in recognizing and classifying cells. Applications have already been demonstrated to the recognition of lymphocytes carrying the HIV virus (Nuovo *et al.*, 1994). Other applications are sure to follow for other important viruses such as Cytomegalovirus (CMV), Epstein–Barr Virus (EBV) and Human Papilloma Virus (HPV). Similar methods will also be applied to the detection of other sequences, especially to the early detection of malignant cells.

One result of the wider use of this technology will be the need for instruments capable of detecting and counting rare cells. As the specificity of the tags increases the number of cells which are tagged will be reduced. Taking the example of HIV it will probably be necessary to exploit the FISH technology to identify one labelled lymphocyte per ten thousand. Cell counters and flow cytometers have difficulty in achieving reliable results at such low counting rates for two related reasons:

1. False triggers resulting from noise pulses exceeding the discriminator thresholds typically occur at rates equivalent to the expected arrival rates for positive cells.
2. There is no ability to verify the presence of the positive cell by recovering it and viewing it under the microscope.

Thus, the use of more specific tags such as the FISH technology will require a new type of cell counter. These systems must have the ability to rapidly interrogate a large field, detect and count the rarely occurring labelled cells. They must also provide the capability to validate positive specimens by visual microscopy.

Several instruments have recently been reported which address this growing need. One device, the Laser Scanning Cytometer (Martin-Reay, 1994), from CompuCyte is clearly designed with this problem in mind. In this instrument, which is based on a microscope, a rapid scan with a

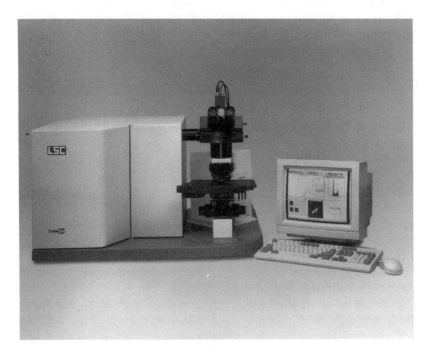

Figure 7.4   Photograph of the LSC Laser Scanning Cytometer. Courtesy of the
CompuCyte corporation, Cambridge, MA, USA

relatively large laser spot is used to locate the target cells. Labelled
cells which are found may be viewed directly or with a CCD camera.
Figure 7.4 is a photograph of the CompuCyte instrument.

Another instrument, which has recently been marketed by Becton
Dickinson as the "DISCOVERY" system, has also been reported
(Schipper *et al.*, 1994) with applications to finding rare cells labelled
specifically (Mesker *et al.*, 1994). Figure 7.5 is a photograph of the
"DISCOVERY" system. This instrument, which was originally developed for cellular research, is also microscope based and has the unique
capability of scanning the image at both high and low resolution simultaneously.

A third instrument, the Chemscan, which is marketed by CHEMU-
NEX has also been reported to have applications to rare event detection
in cell biology (Duquenne *et al.*, 1995). This device which is shown in
Figure 7.6 was developed originally for automation of the Direct Epi-
fluorescence Filter Technique (DEFT) in Microbiology. In the DEFT
analysis a filter membrane is scanned to locate any stained bacteria.

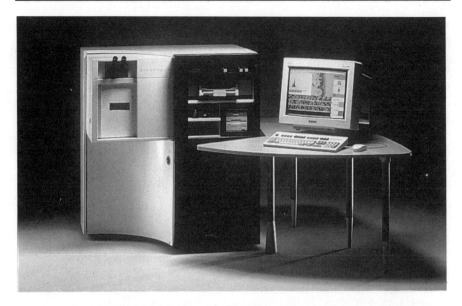

Figure 7.5 Photograph of the DISCOVERY research station. Courtesy of Becton Dickinson Cellular Imaging Systems, Leiden, The Netherlands

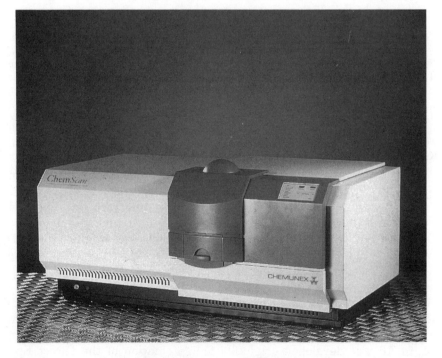

Figure 7.6 Photograph of the Chemscan instrument. Courtesy of Chemunex S.A. Maisons-Alfort, France

Unlike the other two instruments the Chemscan is not microscope based, but provides a rapid scan (2–3 minutes) with an Argon laser of a 25 mm by 25 mm surface to locate labelled particles. The location of the target cells is stored electronically and the specimen may then be transferred to an accessory microscope for visual verification.

It is unlikely that all of the projects described in this chapter will reach successful application in the future hematology laboratory. Some may have limited application in certain laboratories and some remain of only research interest. What is clear, however, is that the hematology laboratory of the future will have greater capabilities for automation and for automated cell classification than presently exists.

REFERENCES

Bull, B.S. and Korpman, R.A. (1978) The logistics of the leukocyte differential count: implications for automation. In Koepke, J.A. (ed.) *Differential Leukocyte Counting*. College of American Pathologists, Skokie, IL.

Davis, G. M. (1994) Auto-verification of the peripheral blood count. *Lab. Med.* **25**: 528.

Duquenne, O., Mignon, K., Butor, C.M. and Guillet, J.-G. (1995) Rare Event Detection in Cell Biology Tumors and Viruses. 7th European Congress on Biotechnology 19:23 Feb.

Hamburger, H.A., McCarthy, R. and Deodhar, S. (1989) Assessment of interlaboratory variability in analytic cytology. *Arch. Pathol. Lab. Med.* **11**: 667–72.

ICSH (1982) Recommendations for the analysis of red cell, white cell and platelet size distribution curves. I. General Principles. *Journal of Clinical Pathol.* **35**: 1320–22.

ICSH (1988) Recommendations for the analysis of red cell, white cell and platelet size distribution curves. II. Methods for fitting a single reference distribution and assessing its goodness of fit. *Clin. Lab. Haematol.* **12**: 417–31.

Kamentsky, L.A. and Kamentsky, L.D. (1991) Microscope-based multiparameter laser scanning cytometer yielding data comparable to flow cytometery data. *Cytometry* **12**: 381–7.

Kasdan, H.L. *et al.* (1994) The white leukocyte differential analyzer for rapid high-precision differentials based on images of cytoprobe reacted cells. *Clin. Chem* **40**(9): 1850–61.

Manian, B.S., Dubrow, R. and Hartz, T. (1994) Volumetric Capillary Cytometry: A new method for absolute cell counts in homogeneous format. (Personal communication).

Martin-Reay, D.G. *et al.* (1994) Evaluation of a new slide-based laser scanning cytometer for DNA analysis of tumors. *Am. J. Clin. Pathol.* **102**; 432–8.

Mesker, W.E., Van der Burg, Oud, P.S., Knepfle, C.F.H.M., Ouwerkerk-van Velsen, M.C.M., Schipper, N.W. and Tanke, H.J. (1994) Detection of immunocytochemically stained rare events using image analysis. *Cytometry* **17**: 209–215.

Metcalf, D. (1994) Thrombopoietin—at last. *Nature* **369**: 519–20.

Nuovo, G.J. *et al.* (1994) In-situ detection of PCR-amplified HIV-1 nucleic acids in lymph nodes and peripheral blood in patients with asymptomatic HIV-1 infection and advanced-stage AIDS. *J. Acquired Immune Deficiency Syndromes* **7**: 916–23.

Ornstein, L. (1993) Hierarchic Heuristic: relevance to economic pattern-recognition and high speed data-processing. Unpublished paper.

Schipper, N.W., Nauwelars, F.A. and Ploem, J.S. (1994) The DISCOVERY system. In Grohs, H.K. and Husain, O.A. (eds) *Automated Cervical Cancer Screening*. Igaku-Shoin, New York, Tokyo. pp 270–78.

Shack, R.V. *et al.* (1987) Design for a fast fluorescence laser scanning microscope. *Anal. Quant. Cytol. Hist.* **9**: 509–20.

Simson, E. (1984) *Hematology Beyond the Microscope*. Technicon Instrument Corp.

Simson, E., Ross, D. and Kocher, W.D. (1988) *Atlas of Automated Cytochemical Hematology*. Technicon Instrument Corp.

Terstappen, W.M.M. *et al.* (1991) Multi-dimensional flow cytometric blood cell differentiation without erythrocyte lysis. *Blood Cells* **17**: 585–602.

FURTHER READING

Drewinko, B. *et al.* (1977) Computerized Hematology. *Am. J. Clin. Pathol.* **67**: 64–76.

Healy, J.C. and Bozek, S.A. (1991) Wright Geimsa: A computer based system for the creation and presentation of peripheral blood smears. *Lab. Med.* **22**(10): 728.

Markin, R.S. and Sasaki, M. (1992) A Laboratory Automation Platform: The Next Robotic Step. MLO, October.

McNeely, M.D. (1982) *Computerized Interpretation of Laboratory Tests: An Overview of Systems, Basic Principles, and Logic Techniques*. 26th Annual National Conference of the Canadian Society of Clinical Chemists.

Siguel, E.N. (1991) *The Future of Computer Aided Diagnosis in the Laboratory*. MLO, August.

Terstappen, W.M.M. and Levin, J. (1992) Bone marrow cell differential counts obtained by multi-dimensional flow cytometery. *Blood Cells* **18**: 311–30.

Index

Note: Page references in *italics* refer to Figures; those in **bold** refer to Tables

Index compiled by Annette Musker